Second Editi

BECOMING INFLUENTIAL

A GUIDE FOR NURSES

Eleanor J. Sullivan, PhD, RN, FAAN

School of Nursing

University of Kansas

Kansas City, Kansas

PEARSON

Boston Columbus Indianapolis New York San Francisco
Upper Saddle River Amsterdam Cape Town Dubai London Madrid
Milan Munich Paris Montreal Toronto Delhi Mexico City
Sao Paulo Sydney Hong Kong Seoul Singapore Taipei Tokyo

Publisher: Julie Levin Alexander
Publisher's Assistant: Regina Bruno
Executive Acquisitions Editor: Pamela Fuller
Editorial Assistant: Cindy Gates
Production Project Manager: Debbie Ryan
Full-Service Project Management: Mohinder Singh/Aptara®, Inc.
Director of Marketing: David Gesell
Marketing Manager: Phoenix Harvey
Marketing Specialist: Michael Sirinides
Art Director: Jayne Conte
Cover Designer: Suzanne Behnke
Cover Art: Fotolia
Composition: Aptara®, Inc.
Printer/Binder: Edwards Brothers Malloy
Cover Printer: Edwards Brothers Malloy
Text Font: ITC Garamond Std Book, 10/12

Credits and acknowledgments borrowed from other sources and reproduced, with permission, in this textbook appear on the appropriate page within text.

Library of Congress Cataloging-in-Publication Data
Sullivan, Eleanor J.,
Becoming influential: a guide for nurses/Eleanor J. Sullivan.—2nd ed.
p. ; cm.
Includes bibliographical references and index.
ISBN-13: 978-0-13-270668-1
ISBN-10: 0-13-270668-7
I. Title.
1. Nursing. 2. Power (Psychology) 3. Career Mobility. 4. Communication.
5. Interpersonal Relations.
LC classification not assigned
610.7306'99—dc23

2011033274

10 9 8 7 6 5

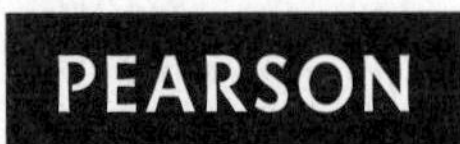

ISBN 10: 0-13-270668-7
ISBN 13: 978-0-13-270668-1

In memory of

Joan Hrubetz, PhD, RN

An influential nurse

BRIEF CONTENTS

BRIEF CONTENTS

CONTENTS

PREFACE

This book is predicated on three assumptions:

1. Nurses, individually and collectively, do not have a history of being influential in health care and other arenas.
2. Although the external environment has contributed to nurses' lack of influence, recent changes in health care portend well for nurses' opportunities to acquire more influence.
3. Nurses can develop the skills to take advantage of these opportunities and become more influential.

This is a presumptuous book. It is presumptuous in assuming that nurses don't have the skills to influence, assuming that they want them, and assuming that I know what these skills are and how to teach them—all brash assumptions. Nonetheless, I am stepping out boldly to proclaim that nurses and nursing could and should be more influential. Culled from years of experience in nursing and from life, I've seen what's worked, what I've done right, what I've done wrong (the best way to learn), and what I've watched others do both right and wrong, relative to the ability to influence. I believe nurses can and should learn these skills to benefit the health and well-being of those in our charge: our current and future patients.

Some of the content presented here is not found elsewhere, and you will find some information here that even your mentors won't tell you. It is hard-hitting, and some of nursing's "sacred cows" are criticized. Do not be put off by this. Use these statements to generate debate in your classes and with your colleagues. Free and open exchange of ideas is the hallmark of an educated profession, and it is my belief that nurses are mature and capable enough to debate our issues without rancor.

This book will not help you pass state boards, prepare you to pass a certifying exam, or improve your clinical skills, per se. What it can do, if you are willing to learn and practice the tools presented here, is help you do your work better and easier, with confidence born of knowledge and the high regard for yourself and your work that you deserve. You will be able to care for your patients; teach your students; interact with superiors, subordinates, and coworkers; and contribute to your profession more fully and in concert with your own abilities.

CHANGES TO THE SECOND EDITION

The second edition of *Becoming Influential: A Guide for Nurses* has been updated with current information on nursing, health care, and technology, including social media. Also added to each chapter are web and print resources and a sidebar especially for the novice nurse.

The book is organized into three parts. Part I, Understanding Influence, covers the basics of power and influence, including how influence works, how to understand and use your power and your image, how to make your interactions more effective, and how you can use politics to be more influential.

Part II, Using Influence, deals with specific strategies to help you become influential, including how to achieve your goals, build a network, work with others to accomplish mutual objectives, become a skilled negotiator, and deal with difficult people and problems.

Part III, Putting Influence to Work, encompasses perfecting your newly acquired skills, telling others about nursing, managing your career, and balancing your life.

Part IV, The Final Steps, explains how to prepare your successors and leave your legacy.

An appendix lists ten little-known secrets of success.

Some content you already know and use often. Other content may be new to you, or you may have wondered how some people seem to be more effective in getting their ideas implemented. If so, this book's for you.

I have often thought that the world of work is somehow not real life. Real life consisted of friends and families, work and play, good times and bad. That, I know now, is both true and false. Work consists of life and relationships, but it is not all of life. It is a part of our lives and one that plays a large part in our daily existence and in the way we see ourselves now and into the future. Work is important but not the only important aspect of ourselves.

In work, as in life, we are always becoming. We are never finished growing, developing, and changing. So it is in becoming influential. But know one thing: you are becoming the best that you can be.

Good luck!

ACKNOWLEDGMENTS

As always, no writer creates a book alone. Colleagues and friends have shared ideas, information, and experiences over the years; many of those suggestions have found their way into this book. A special thanks to pioneers in helping foster nurses' influence, including nurses Melodie Chenevert and Marie Manthey and non-nurse Jinx Melia. Readers today have the advantage of knowledge culled from these experts.

Editor Pamela Fuller and her assistant, Cynthia Gates, along with the staff at Pearson Health Science, have made creating this book easier and its content better than the author could have imagined.

Reviewers' careful reading also found critical and troublesome parts and made thoughtful suggestions to improve the manuscript. To all the nurses who've shared their wisdom with me, I thank you.

Eleanor J. Sullivan, PhD, RN, FAAN

Reviewers

Thank You

My heartfelt thanks go out to my colleagues from schools of nursing across the country who have given their time generously to help me create this exciting new edition of *Becoming Influential*. I have reaped the benefit of your collective experience as nurses and teachers, and I have made many improvements thanks to your efforts. Among those who gave us their encouragement and comments are:

Michael Barbour, RN, MSN
Professor
Florida State University
Panama City, Florida

Sharon E. Beck, PhD, RN
Independent Contractor/Consultant
Laguna Woods, California

Gail Bromley, PhD, RN
Associate Dean, Academics
Kent State University
Kent, Ohio

Mary Camann, PhD, PMHCNS-BC
Associate Professor
Kennesaw State University
Kennesaw, Georgia

Janet B. Craig, MSN, MBA, DHA, RN, CENP
Associate Professor,
Extramural Program Officer
Clemson University
Clemson, South Carolina

Deborah L. Dalrymple, RN, MSN, CRNI
Professor
Montgomery County Community College
Blue Bell, Pennsylvania

Susan B. del Bene, PhD, RN, CNS
Associate Professor
Pace University
New York, New York

Gloria Fowler, MN, RN
Clinical Assistant Professor, Director of Student Affairs
University of South Carolina
Columbia, South Carolina

Lucille Gambardella, PhD, APN-BC, CNE, ANEF
Chair/Professor and Director of Graduate Programs
Wesley College
Dover, Delaware

Alice Kempe, PhD, CS
Associate Professor
Ursuline College
Pepper Pike, Ohio

Tammie McCoy, RN, PhD
Professor and Department Chair
Mississippi University for Women
Columbus, Mississippi

ABOUT THE AUTHOR

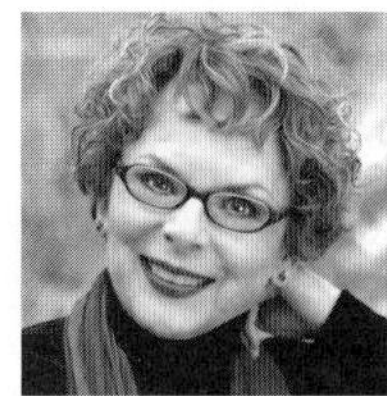

Eleanor J. Sullivan, PhD, RN, is the former dean of the University of Kansas School of Nursing, past president of Sigma Theta Tau International, and a previous editor of the *Journal of Professional Nursing*. She has served on the board of directors of the American Association of Colleges of Nursing and on an advisory council at the National Institutes of Health, among other professional positions. Dr. Sullivan is known for her publications in nursing, including her award-winning textbook *Effective Leadership and Management in Nursing*, soon to be released in its eighth edition, as well as numerous articles in nursing and health care publications.

In addition to her books for nurses, Dr. Sullivan also writes mystery novels, the first three featuring nurses (*Twice Dead*, *Deadly Diversion*, *Assumed Dead*). Her latest book, *Cover Her Body*, *A Singular Village Mystery,* is the first in a new series of historical mysteries featuring a nineteenth-century midwife. Other books in the series will soon follow.

Connect with her at http://www.EleanorSullivan.com and on LinkedIn and Facebook.

ABOUT THE AUTHOR

PART I

Understanding Influence

1

What Is Influence and Why Do I Need It?

No one can make you feel inferior without your consent.

ELEANOR ROOSEVELT

In this chapter, you will learn:

- What influence is
- What barriers impede nurses from being as influential as they could be
- How nursing's influence is poised to improve
- Why you need influence
- What you risk becoming influential
- How to become influential

INFLUENCE DEFINED

Influence is relative in that it is related to a specified goal within the context of your own life and work. A person may have influence at work but not in the community, or vice versa—or he or she may have influence in both. One is influential to the extent that he or she is able to communicate ideas to others and gain their support through acceptance or participation. Thus, influence exists only in relationships with others.

Influence is more important than authority. You are wise to use influence instead of authority, or at least before you use authority—as anyone who has ever dealt with a teenager knows. Influence is affected by everything about you, personally and professionally.

Influence can be bestowed, as in winning an election or being appointed a nurse manager, or earned as a result of respect for your work. Expert nurses have influence, for example, because of their knowledge and skill. Influence can be limited, such as at work, or can be broader, encompassing a community, state, nation, or the world. Sometimes a person becomes influential as a result of overcoming incredible odds or after a lifetime of accomplishments. Nelson Mandela is influential, for instance, because of the contributions he made to ending apartheid in South Africa.

Influence can fluctuate as events unfold. Politicians often become less influential as stories of their personal behavior become public. Others become more influential if they establish popular programs, receive awards, or accomplish notable feats such as climbing Mt. Everest. Influence can deteriorate or even vanish if a well-regarded person is convicted of committing a crime, or, conversely, becomes more popular because of the notoriety. (Celebrities are in this category.)

Influence cannot be bought (not easily, anyway), sold, bartered, or even thrown away. It cannot be held in your hand, put up on a wall, or hidden under a barrel. It can be earned through effort; most important, *the skills of influence can be taught and learned*, not unlike the way we learn clinical skills. Making a decision to become influential is the first, necessary step to gaining influence.

For the Novice Nurse

You're beginning a fascinating and rewarding career, and this book will help you. Little of this content was included in your course work; it was not covered in clinical experiences, either. But don't despair. You're in luck. In the following chapters, you'll discover everything you've ever wanted to know about what happens in the real world.

Ready? Go!

BARRIERS TO NURSING'S INFLUENCE

Barriers to nursing's influence come from both the external world and inside the profession itself. Let's examine several of these.

External Barriers

The *structure of the health care system* has been a consistent barrier to nursing's influence. This structure has allowed physicians, health care administrators, and third-party payers (e.g., insurance companies, Medicare) to control funding for health care and thus the ability to ration who gets what care, where, when, and from whom. (See the section "The (Really) Good News" later in this chapter on how change is coming.)

Another barrier to nursing's influence has been the public's long-standing and *inaccurate perception of nurses and the work they do.* People are seldom aware of the level of skill or education required to be a knowledgeable and competent nurse unless they have experienced extensive nursing care or observed such care given to a family member.

ON THE OTHER HAND. Despite reports of medical mistakes, denial of care by insurers, and the high cost of prescription drugs—all of which have tarnished the image of health care in general—the public's trust in nurses continues to be high. As they have in previous years, nurses continue to be rated highest among all professions in honesty and ethical standards (Gallup, 2010a). In addition, the Gallup organization found that leaders in government, industry, universities, and health services believe that nurses reduce medical errors and improve patient safety and that they should have more influence in health care (Gallup, 2010b).

Furthermore, nursing has emerged as a discipline with a credible scientific base, as evidenced by its government-funded support through the National Institute of Nursing Research at the National Institutes of Health (NIH). The concerted efforts by nursing organizations and the lobbying of many individual nurses resulted in creation of the National Center for Nursing Research at NIH in the mid-1980s, which Congress passed over President Reagan's veto. (The National Center for Nursing Research later became the National Institute of Nursing Research.) This is an excellent example of influence that can and should be brought to bear to advance nursing's agenda for improving health care.

Nurse leaders are cited in *Modern Healthcare*'s 2010 list of the 100 most powerful people in health care, including Beverly Malone (National League for Nursing chief executive officer), Rebecca Patton (American Nurses Association president), and Linda Aiken (renowned authority on nurse staffing) (Vesely, 2010).

Nurses also hold influential positions in government. Seven nurses serve in the 112th U.S. Congress. Mary Wakefield heads the Health Resources and Services Administration in the U.S. Department of Health and Human Services. Patricia Grady leads the National Institute of Nursing Research at NIH. Clara Adams-Ender rose to the rank of Brigadier General in the U.S. Army and became the first black woman to command an Army post. But, like women CEOs in Fortune 500 companies, they are few in comparison to the number of men in influential positions (Lantz, 2008).

Internal Barriers

The culture of the nursing profession reflects its historical roots from military, religious, and women's history as well as that of a repressed people. That is, nurses tend to downplay achievements: their own and those of other nurses. Nursing educators who teach doctoral students have seen their share of students who seem to continually undo their good work, leading many to wonder if the students' colleagues or spouses have discouraged them to the point where they actually sabotage their own efforts, thereby maintaining an illusion that the program was just too difficult for them.

Even nurses who become successful as skilled clinicians or community leaders, for example, often are caught diminishing their own accomplishments. This problem happens often enough that we must wonder whether the culture of nursing has discouraged success. The term "one-woman show"—often heard when a nurse reports an accomplishment, such as an article in a professional journal—is in itself telling, as if doing something on one's own is somehow acting phony or being a show-off. (See how one nurse dealt with a problem she experienced when practicing influence in the Chapter 10 case study.)

Nurses also may sabotage their effectiveness in even more subtle ways. Anecdotes abound about nurses' lack of support for each other, with nurses accused of "eating their own." This situation is not unlike reports that women do not support other women in business. If society does not value nurses and their work, is it any wonder that nurses themselves do not respect each other?

Finally, nursing is not easily explained. The work is intimate, messy, and deals with multiple facets of individuals' lives, bodies, and illnesses. When talking about our work, nurses have tended to focus on the *process* of care (the nature of nursing work) rather than the *outcome* of their work. That focus has changed in recent times, however, as funding has become tied to outcomes, and all health care providers have been forced to be increasingly accountable for the outcomes, as well as the costs, of their work. The outcome of nursing is the patient's improvement, adjustment to changed circumstances, or dignified death; nothing could be more valuable to the individuals who entrust us with their care.

THE (REALLY) GOOD NEWS

Nursing's access to patients promises to improve. With the passage of health care reform legislation, nurses stand to gain influence in several ways (Stokowski, 2010). The Patient Protection and Affordable Care Act (PPACA), signed into law on March 23, 2010, is prevention- and community-oriented legislation. It provides funding for both advanced nursing practice and general nursing education, expansion of primary care into school-based clinics, nurse-managed clinics, home care support, transitional care, and a service corps for rural areas. Acute care settings, too, will see an increase in patient numbers as previously uninsured patients access needed care.

The Institute of Medicine's (IOM) report on the future of nursing makes sweeping recommendations for nursing's future, including that "nurses should be full partners, with physicians and other health care professionals, in redesigning health care in the United States" (Institute of Medicine, 2010, p. 3). In addition, the Carnegie Foundation recommends radically transforming nursing education (Benner, Sutphen, Leonard, &

Day, 2009). The PPACA bill is only beginning to be implemented, and its regulations have yet to be publicized. Along with the legislation, the IOM report, the Carnegie Foundation's recommendations, and the public's desperate need for health care combine to portend nursing's potential influence in health care for the future.

WHY BE INFLUENTIAL?

Popular literature on power and influence, most often aimed at women, peddles techniques for gaining clout for one's own gain, usually to rise to the top in one's field. Although nurses might achieve success for themselves as they become influential, they have a larger goal—one beyond themselves—which is to be more effective in what they do and to influence health care. Improved patient care, better working conditions for nurses, and better health for people are just a few of the reasons for nurses to develop their skills of influence.

Nurses are influential at the bedside, and they can be influential in any number of other arenas. Formal and informal meetings at work, on committees, in casual conversations, in the community, at professional meetings, and in volunteer groups are among the many opportunities nurses have to be influential. Your identity as a nurse goes with you wherever you are, regardless of whether you are aware of it. How we present ourselves is an outward expression of our inner experience. Our beliefs about ourselves color all that we do and say.

BECOMING INFLUENTIAL

Presenting Yourself

The first step to becoming influential is to assess the way you present yourself (Pagana, 2010). Self-presentation includes subtle and not-so-subtle behaviors along with appearance (yes, appearance does matter). It originates with your attitude about yourself. Do you see yourself as an accomplished professional? Do you believe your colleagues are as well? Do you think your attitude is reflected in the way you present yourself?

The next step is to evaluate your current ability to be influential. Use feedback from others, either formal (such as performance evaluations) or informal (such as when friends or colleagues offer compliments or observations). Most important is your assessment of your own skills of influence. This appraisal should be ongoing; continually evaluate how effective certain strategies are with various individuals and groups until you have a good sense of how to respond in a variety of situations.

Developing a desired self-presentation is needed to improve your ability to be effective in meeting your goals and those of nursing. The following chapters will help you learn how to understand and develop this and other skills and will help you deal with difficult and challenging problems and issues.

Can you imagine the magnitude of nursing's influence if all nurses learned these skills?

THE RISKS OF BECOMING INFLUENTIAL

All opportunities come with risk, including opportunities for influence. Any action with the potential for success comes with an equal opportunity for failure. The effects of powerful medications—with their potential to heal, as well as the possibility of harm—serve as examples.

One risk is inspiring envy and jealousy. (Who does she think she is?) Another is differentiating yourself from others. (She's changed.) Raised expectations is another. (I thought he would do better.)

Conversely, the opportunities to influence nursing care, to provide direction for organizations, and to contribute to change for the future exist as well.

Influence is like money; we seldom have too much.

What You Know Now

Having studied this first chapter, you have learned that influence exists in your relationships with others. Using influence, you know that you can improve patient care, promote the nursing profession, and enhance the health care environment. You know that there are many barriers, both historically and today, that interfere with nurses' ability to be influential. You have decided that you want to become more influential. You have considered how you present yourself and assessed your ability to influence. You know, too, that there are risks inherent in becoming more influential, and you have decided that you are willing to accept the risks as well as the opportunity to help your patients and your profession. In the following chapters, you will discover many ways to assess and improve your self-presentation on the way to becoming influential.

You are ready to learn more!

Tools for Influence

1. Keep in mind that you can become influential and that the skills to become influential can be learned.
2. What are your motives for improving your ability to influence others? Be honest.
3. Becoming influential has as much to do with attitude as it does with behavior; both are necessary.
4. Recognize the risks inherent in becoming more influential. Accept them.
5. Observe others who are influential, and try to incorporate their behaviors into your repertoire of skills.

Learning Activities

1. Recall three influential people you knew in the past. Why were they influential? Was it due to their position, their personality, or their accomplishments?

   Name three influential people whom you know now. What do they do (as compared to who they are) that makes them influential? For the next week, try incorporating some of their actions into your behavior. Evaluate how easy or difficult that was and how effective you were. Try the same activity the following week.
2. Recall a situation in which you could have been more influential. Write down who was there and what happened. Who had the most influence? Why? What could you have done or said to have more influence?

   Share your experience in class or with a friend. See what you can learn from others' experiences also. Save your notes for Chapter 5.
3. Hold a debate about nurses becoming more influential. Have one person or group claim that nurses should be influential and the other side explain what can go wrong. Think of reasons not included in the chapter.
4. Assess three people in your workplace or classes whom you consider influential. Describe why and how they are influential.

References

Benner, P., Sutphen, M., Leonard, V., & Day, L. (2009). *Educating nurses: A call for radical transformation.* San Francisco: Jossey-Bass.

Gallup. (2010a). Nursing leadership from bedside to boardroom: Opinion leaders' perceptions. Retrieved October 15, 2010, from http://www.rwjf.org/files/research/nursinggalluppolltopline.pdf

Gallup. (2010b). In U.S., more than 8 in 10 rate nurses, doctors highly. Retrieved January 20, 2011, from http://www.gallup.com/poll/145214/Rate-Nurses-Doctors-Highly.aspx

Institute of Medicine (2010). *The future of nursing: Leading change, advancing health.* Retrieved from October 15, 2010, from http://www.thefutureofnursing.org/IOM-Report

Lantz, P. M. (2008). Gender and leadership in healthcare administration: 21st century progress and challenges. *Journal of Healthcare and Management, 53*(5), 291–301.

Pagana, K. D. (2010). 7 tips to improve your professional etiquette. *Nursing Management, 41*(5), 45–48.

Stokowski, L. A. (2010). Healthcare reform and nurses: Challenges and opportunities. *Medscape,* May 6, 2010. Retrieved October 15, 2010, from http://www.medscape.com/viewarticle/721049

Vesely, R. (2010). The 100 most powerful people in healthcare. *Modern Healthcare, 40*(34), 6–7, 24–34.

Web Resources

Sellers, A. (2011). Nursing influence: Topics that influence nurses and the influence nurses have on the community. Retrieved April 15, 2011, from http://nursinginfluence.com

Sullivan, E. J. Ask a nurse. *Journal of Professional Nursing, 17*(5). Retrieved April 14, 2011 from http://www.eleanorsullivan.com/pdf/askanurse.pdf

Sullivan, E. J. Taking the mystery out of influence. Retrieved April 15, 2011 from http://www.eleanorsullivan.com/pdf/Taking_the_Mystery_Out_of_Influence.pdf

Print Resources

Axelrod, A. (2000). *Elizabeth I, CEO: Strategic lessons from the leader who built an empire.* Paramus, NJ: Prentice Hall.

Gerber, R. (2002). *Leadership the Eleanor Roosevelt way: Timeless strategies from the first lady of courage.* New York: Prentice Hall.

2

Rules of the Game

I'd like to make a motion that we accept reality.

Bob Newhart from the *Bob Newhart Show*

In this chapter, you will learn:

- Why work is a game
- What the rules are
- What gender has to do with the rules
- How organizations function
- Why nursing and the rules differ
- How to make the rules work for you

WHAT IS THE GAME?

In the beginning, according to author Jinx Melia's classic book *Breaking into the Boardroom* (1986), survival was the goal. When people lived in caves, she suggests, men went out to hunt for bears and women stayed home and cared for their young. Men competed among themselves for the most attractive and fertile female, but they left those competitions behind when they went out to hunt because they soon learned that they couldn't capture the bear on their own; they needed each other's help. Men established the first political system when they learned to work together to capture the bear. Women, on the other hand, learned to control their environment (the home) and to rely on men for food and protection.

Fast forward to the 21st century. Women have rightfully demanded access to education and to compete with men for positions in any field. At the same time, according to Melia, women expected to continue to be able to control their environment. Here's an example:

> A group of nursing school administrators and faculty leaders were asked by the university's provost to meet with him and discuss use of a conference room in the building the school shared with other health care professions. The conference room was in the section of the building assigned to nursing. The provost explained some changes that had occurred and that he needed to use the conference room for his own office. Although the school had ample conference room space and the room being discussed was seldom used, the nursing faculty (all women) adamantly refused to agree to let the provost use the room. No amount of discussion or even the reality that they did not "own" the space could persuade them from this entrenched position.
>
> Of course, the inevitable happened.
>
> The provost took over the space for his office and mentally dismissed the nursing faculty as not being team players. He would not approach them in the future to participate in mutually-beneficial activities. He, in effect, wrote them off as participants in the health sciences division of the university.

What did these faculty members miss? *They passed up an opportunity to bargain with the provost for something else they wanted*, such as equipment for the skills lab or increased funding for doctoral fellowships. He may not have been able to grant their request, but he would have recognized his debt to them, which they could have cashed sometime in the future. Savvy game players know how to use someone else's request for assistance to gain something for themselves.

For the Novice Nurse

You may think these rules don't apply to you. You know your job—that's all that matters. You couldn't be more wrong. Although it may be the first time you've heard about many of these rules, you'll find that organizations function with them in place.

Ignore them at your peril.

Survival in today's world means success on the job. In nursing, success can be measured by your ability to care for patients, to teach students, or to manage a designated unit, department, or school—and how good you feel about doing the work. You also might measure success by how much you are learning, how you are developing relationships with colleagues to get your work done, and how many contacts you are making to help you in the future. These are all reasonable goals, but—as Melia would argue—women often do not think of them.

Nurses (and many women) tend to think that because we have good intentions (we do), do good work (we do), and are good people (we are), we should be rewarded with money, gratitude, and respect, at the least. When that does not happen, we think there is something wrong with us or with our profession. In reality, we're operating outside the rules.

The rules require the give and take of diplomacy, consideration of contingencies, and allowances for extenuating circumstances. The business of health care is a perfect example of a fluid, changing system requiring flexibility, resourcefulness, and resiliency from its participants. Nurses who want everything to stay the same (to control their environment) have had a sorry awakening in recent times.

WHAT ARE THE RULES?

"Business is a game," says former CNN executive Gail Evans (2003, p. 178). Like all games, there are rules for playing and winning. The rules are not written anywhere. You can't look them up on the Internet. They aren't found in any policy and procedures manual, and you won't learn them in orientation. No matter how skilled you are, if you don't know the rules, you can't play the game.

The object of most games is to reach the goal and to overcome or eliminate obstacles in the way; as in football, the person with the ball is probably going to be tackled. It is this willingness to surmount obstacles and to be tackled that distinguishes a winning player. Those who huddle on the sidelines, worrying about getting hit, are never going to catch the ball—much less score.

> A student came into an advisor's office one day to inquire about the school's graduate programs. He was clearly interested in applying, but he seemed hesitant. The advisor asked him what was wrong. He replied that he didn't know if he would be admitted. His undergraduate grades weren't that good, he admitted, even though they had improved when he had entered the nursing major. He said he thought he better wait and take some courses to bring his grade point average up.
>
> The advisor thought a moment and then she told him, "I can guarantee you one thing." Surprised, the student asked what that was. "If you don't apply," she said, staring him in the eye, "you won't get in." The student submitted his application and was admitted to the graduate program the next fall.

The Basic Rules

Bartering, quid pro quo, the grapevine, nonconfrontational tactics, leverage, losing the battle to win the war, making connections, accepting responsibility, becoming team players, loyalty, seeking mentors, and accepting risk are skills that those with influence have learned (see Table 2-1). Nurses can learn them too.

TABLE 2-1 The Game Rules

Learn to barter	Make connections
Recognize quid pro quo	Accept responsibility
Use the grapevine	Become a team player
Use nonconfrontational tactics	Cultivate loyalty
Use leverage	Seek mentors
Be willing to lose a battle to win a war	Accept risk

LEARN TO BARTER. Exchanging favors is the result of bartering. It's that simple. You do something for me; I'll do something for you. The terms of the exchange may be negotiated informally—"I'll work this weekend for you if you'll work Thanksgiving for me"—or formally, such as in a union contract.

There are many variations in bartering. A nurse who wants a colleague to work the weekend as a favor may not want to work Thanksgiving in return. He or she might say, "I can't work Thanksgiving, but how about New Year's Eve?" This exchange might go back and forth a few times until both parties think that they have made a good bargain.

Often the favor asked does not include a specified return. "I'll work this weekend for you," leaves the person receiving the favor in debt to the one who did the favor once the deal is struck. When the favor-giver asks for something in the future, the debtor is obligated to fulfill it.

The two most important points to remember are: (1) don't ask for a favor without realizing you'll owe in return and (2) when you are asked for a favor, be sure to remember that you are owed. "I'll work for you this weekend, and I'll be sure to ask you sometime when I need a weekend off," is an example of letting the other person know that he owes you.

RECOGNIZE QUID PRO QUO. Bartering is the method; quid pro quo describes the currency. It is the compensation given in return for a favor, product, or service. The currency is also known as chips.

The compensation usually is something the recipient of the initial favor is uniquely qualified to give, such as an introduction to an influential person. The arrangement is similar to purchasing a car or cleaning service for your house except that products and services are usually paid for with money in some form. Quid pro quo is compensation that money cannot buy, for example, the introduction mentioned previously.

Quid pro quo is what you use when your teenager wants to borrow your car. You agree, on the condition that she mow the lawn. You have used what your teenager wants (access to the car) to gain something you want (the lawn mowed).

USE THE GRAPEVINE. The least valuable currency for bartering in business is money; the most valuable is information. Every organization has an informal system of information and communication. It is known as the *grapevine* or the *rumor mill*. Rumors are not exact information; they undergo subtle changes as they are repeated, but essential ideas are retained. Information spread through the grapevine can be acquired only in this way because of the silent conspiracy of employees who keep such information from their superiors in large or small organizations. Access to the grapevine is essential for anyone interested in influence, especially those in management or those who aspire to management positions.

You can be both a source for grapevine information and a receiver of it. People at the lowest level in the organizational hierarchy have the most to gain from knowing what is really going on in the organization. They can barter that information for help they need now or in the future.

If you have a higher-level position, a trusted subordinate or colleague can tell you what is being spread through the grapevine. You, in turn, owe a debt to that person. You may pay with the collegial relationship you two share or, more often, you will be called to pay by supporting the person for a promotion, for example. Regardless, the debt is worth it because there is no other way to find out this information, especially before it is made public.

USE NONCONFRONTATIONAL TACTICS. Another word for nonconfrontational tactics (a term used erroneously by people who are not savvy about the rules) is manipulation. Direct confrontation is rarely effective. It often results in both parties digging into entrenched positions. Stalemate over a union contract is an example.

The long-running television show *M*A*S*H* illustrated numerous examples of nonconfrontational tactics as well as the less-successful use of power. The least powerful person in the unit, the company clerk, was successful because he repeatedly steered the commander into doing what was best for the unit. The chief nurse, who had considerably more power than the clerk, was often heavy-handed in dealing with the commander, and the consequences were frequently less effective.

USE LEVERAGE. Leverage is the power that one person has to achieve a desired outcome. The power may not really exist, but "perception is truth," according to a marketing adage. Your boss has leverage. She can discipline you, transfer you, or fire you. Or can she? If you think she can, then she can. Your boss's leverage is likely to be real; other forms of leverage are less obvious.

Political situations offer numerous examples of the use of leverage. Countries or individuals believed to have nuclear weapons have leverage over those that do not. The proverbial "line in the sand" illustrates the use of leverage: cross the line and suffer the consequences. Often, there are no consequences because the person issuing the challenge cannot or will not do anything in response. The person is bluffing. He is counting on you believing that he will do something. That's his power.

LOSE THE BATTLE TO WIN THE WAR. Sometimes it is advisable to lose a battle; the payoff may help you win the war. The battle is an individual incident, and the war is the long-term outcome. Military strategists have long recognized the value of losing one battle to take more ground in another place. That is the reason to deploy forces in various strategic locations and is similar to buying both stocks and bonds to allow for wins to counteract loses.

Sometimes even winning the battle is not what it seems. Remember the faculty group who refused to budge on allowing the university provost to acquire their conference room for his office? They stuck to their principles, or so they thought. In reality, they lost both the battle and the war.

The question to ask is: What will I gain if I lose or give up this battle? Is it worth it in the long term? "I want to attend the class on advanced cardiac care next week," the new staff nurse said to her supervisor, who argued that she didn't think the staff nurse was proficient enough yet to benefit from the class. The staff nurse insisted and—having no one else requesting the same class—the supervisor relented. The staff nurse won the battle, but her supervisor learned that she had a staff member who was inflexible and demanding. When other opportunities arose in the future, this staff nurse would be less likely to be selected.

MAKE CONNECTIONS. Who you know, rather than what you know, is still true. So how do you meet the people who can help you and influence your future? You can take advantage of an opportunity—for example, introduce yourself to a speaker at a conference—or you may be introduced through another person in the course of a business or social event. Another way is to ask someone directly to introduce you in person or online through social media, such as LinkedIn or Facebook.

The secret to connecting with people you want to meet is small talk (Baber & Waymon, 2007). Small talk sounds miniscule and unimportant; it is neither. It is the social lubricant by which people form and keep relationships. It is as valuable as—or possibly more valuable than—online communication. Your networks of people you can help and who can help you are developed this way. (You will learn more about small talk and other communication strategies throughout this book.)

Brokering people (bartering connections) benefits all the players. When you introduce two people with mutual interests, you may profit from the connection as well if the introduction serves them both. Now they both owe you. The opportunities are infinite for all the people involved—those introducing, the people being introduced, and the individual with a stated agenda. Networks are formed just this way. You can do it too.

ACCEPT RESPONSIBILITY. Acknowledging and avoiding responsibility are two sides to the same matter but with very different results. Accepting responsibility does not mean just acknowledging blame; it can and should be used to take credit and collect a debt (see the section "Recognize quid pro quo" earlier in this chapter).

Avoiding responsibility, on the other hand, sometimes becomes a career goal of people without power. "I didn't do it," claims the child staring at crayon marks on the wall. "The computer did it," the clerk says with a shrug.

Individuals in many situations and at all levels of an organization attempt to avoid responsibility, especially when something might go wrong. This tactic is known as CYA (Cover Your A__). "The patient *appeared* to be sleeping" strikes most people as ludicrous when loud snores are coming from the patient's room. Nurses commonly write such a statement and similar ones in the nurses' notes to protect themselves in case it is later found out that the patient was awake, although it's unclear what the consequences of that finding would be.

When things go wrong in an organization, it is most often a system failure. Medical mistakes—found to be so numerous that a report of them sparked a vigorous public outcry, a demand for corrections, and revised Medicare reimbursement regulations—are a result of failure in the system of delivering care. Multiple individuals and the system under which they work are to blame.

In today's litigious society, however, it is unsurprising that people are reluctant to accept responsibility for a mistake serious enough to harm someone. Regardless, accepting the problem and crafting a solution is a challenge demanded of professionals in the health care system. On an individual level, approaching a problematic situation with the goal to correct it and—more important—to avoid the same occurrence in the future is the best way to handle mistakes. No one is perfect: not even nurses. Just be careful to whom and how you report a mistake. Separating blame and discipline from incident reporting is one way to encourage staff to report negative events (Sullivan, 2013). Then changes, if needed, can be identified and implemented.

BECOME A TEAM PLAYER. Playing on teams began with the bear hunt. No hunter could be successful alone. Nor would he necessarily survive. Individuals give up some of their own independence to work for the good of the team. In the end, the team hopes to win, which makes all the players winners. Certain rules govern team play. They include:

Never attack your own members.

Don't sabotage your side's strategy.

Follow the leader.

Your results rest on the actions of everyone on the team.

Defeat just means defeat of today's game; you can play another game tomorrow.

If you don't like how the team plays, go elsewhere.

CULTIVATE LOYALTY. Loyalty is the attribute most valued by influential people, but loyalty means different things to different people. To a game player, one who operates within the rules, loyalty means doing whatever the team leader says *while the game is being played*. When the game is over (i.e., negotiation completed), loyalties can change. Other people (Melia suggests these include women who are not savvy) think loyalty means forever, much like marriage. The problem, Melia says, comes with the conditions that long-term loyalty implies. These are inappropriate for work, where loyalties can and do shift with the issue being considered (Melia, 1986).

If you accept a job, you owe your employer your loyalty while you are on the job. Your debt includes showing up, suiting up, and doing the job. You also promise (though it's not in writing) to keep your boss informed about anything that he or she needs to know and to support your boss's decisions to internal and external publics. That is, you don't have to agree with your boss in private, but don't criticize the decision when talking with your colleagues. Also, don't let your boss be surprised about anything that could be harmful if you learn it first.

> Two nurses were overheard in the cafeteria talking about their boss. No matter what was said, such a conversation was inappropriate in a public place. In another instance, an assistant complained to the patient about how much she disliked her job while she was bathing him.

Loyalty is a form of quid pro quo. Once you agree to do a job or support a cause, you are obligated to deliver. If you agree to support a proposal that a colleague is planning to present at an upcoming committee meeting, for example, you must be loyal to that commitment. You cannot go behind the colleague's back and tell people otherwise. This rule does not mean that you cannot change your mind when you receive more information. Once that issue is settled, however, you are free to give your loyalty to other people and situations.

SEEK MENTORS. Mentoring in nursing has become more commonplace, with both potential mentors and mentees recognizing the value of the relationship (Grossman, 2007). Nonetheless, game players realize that they must find mentors to support their professional growth. You may think that your work should speak for itself—that if you do a good enough job, a higher-level person will see what you can do and offer to help you. That is seldom the case. It is your job to cultivate possible mentors.

You can find mentors among the people in your own organization who have positions at a level higher than yours. You can have more than one mentor, and mentors can be nurses or come from other disciplines. You also can find mentors among members of professional associations in nursing and related professions, such as a local hospital association.

A mentor is someone whose words, behaviors, and style you admire. You may not agree with everything a mentor does, but you recognize this person as someone who could teach you. Similarly, the mentor expresses some interest in you and your work. Often, a supervisor will serve as a mentor. The mentor-mentee relationship might not even be named as such. You might realize that you go to the person for advice or that this person has been a special help to you.

Mentoring is a power relationship of *equal support* between two persons of unequal rank. You have as much responsibility to the mentor as he or she does to you. Protection from adverse consequences is what you and your mentor exchange. Because the mentee is in a lower-level position, either in the same organization or a similar one in the industry, the mentee has access to information via the grapevine that the mentor who is at a higher level in the organization would not. By the same token, the mentor often has knowledge that could help the mentee (e.g., job openings before they are announced, a change in the organization's mission) and would be able to alert the mentee to these opportunities.

The mentor also is essential in furthering your career outside of the organization by, for example, introducing you to key people in a professional association, suggesting your name for important committees, or nominating you for positions. The mentor is available for advice and counsel as your career moves along. In return, you have a career-long obligation to support and protect the mentor, especially publicly.

> At one hospital, the rumor mill had it that the chief nurse, who was a mentor to a nurse manager, was about to be fired. The nurse manager was conflicted. Should she continue to support her boss to her colleagues and her staff? If she did, would she be fired too? Or miss out on chances for promotion in the future? If she didn't support her boss, would she be seen as disloyal and not be trusted in the future? Using the principles of the mentor-mentee relationship just described, what do you think she should do? (See activity 3 at the end of the chapter.)

Another obligation is to repay your mentor by publicly recognizing your mentor when you have achieved a level of success. Academy Award winners thanking people is an example. Graduate students often become mentees of their advisors, who help them with their careers long after the students have finished school. When the student publishes a paper from a thesis or dissertation, the faculty member may be included as a second author, if appropriate, or acknowledged in print.

ACCEPT RISK. Taking chances in the modern world is safe compared to the world the bear hunters experienced when they left the cave. We, of course, can be in danger when we pull out onto a highway, submit to a surgical procedure, or are simply at the wrong place at the wrong time. We accept the risk in order to live our lives, and most of the time we do that without excessive fear. (Unfortunately, terrorists' acts have reminded us that everyday life can assume monumental danger.)

The risks that most of us try to avoid are failure and its resulting humiliation. The consequences of public failure are so embarrassing that some people will do almost anything to avoid the possibility of failure. The flip side of failure, though, is success. As we learned from the student who was reluctant to apply to graduate school, if we don't take a risk (in his case, by applying to graduate school), we also don't have the chance of success.

How many nurses do you know who would never consider going to another institution to work? Or applying for a different job in their own organization? Why? Because they might not be able to do the job or they might not like the new boss? What do you think they might be missing because they aren't willing to risk failure?

Influential people risk failure regularly. Politicians who run for office risk failure. The nurse who proposes a new model for arranging care for at-risk newborns risks failure. Successful people have failures; unsuccessful people rarely do. Why? Because they don't take a risk. What else do they risk? Success! If you decide you want to be more influential than you are, you must decide how much of a risk you are willing to take.

Remember: being embarrassed is not fatal.

The Game Board

Whatever game you play includes a game board or a playing field, whether it's Scrabble® or soccer. The same is true in business. You wouldn't try to play Clue® on a Monopoly® board or baseball on a football field. But that is just what people do if they don't know the game of business.

The traditional playing field in business is a triangle with the most people along the base and the fewest at the top. There is a strict chain of command, and everyone knows who's in charge. Problem solving may be less successful and creativity may be stifled because fewer people are involved at the highest levels of decision making.

Women, however, tend to want the game board to be a circle so that everyone is included. In this model, everyone gets heard and no one gets above anyone else. Problem solving and creativity improves, but the group may be unable to come to a decision and movement upward may be thwarted.

This interest in a circular design may help explain why nurses seem reluctant to support the work of other nurses. A nurse entrepreneur reported on her lack of success in selling prints of her nursing artwork to other nurses. "Why should she make money off us?" the entrepreneur overheard one nurse say. Why not? Framed prints depicting nursing in an interesting and positive way could help nurses celebrate their own work as well as help the public and future potential students view nursing accurately.

On the other hand, shared governance is a popular organizational arrangement in many health care institutions (McDowell et al., 2010). Shared governance allows individual members of the organization, especially those directly involved in the service provided, to make decisions collectively and to be accountable for those decisions. Shared governance takes advantage of nurses' contact with their patients and with each other and of their knowledge of the best way to deliver care. A variety of organizational models are being developed as health care is evolving in response to the health care reform legislation, expanding technology, and increasing medical advances.

GENDER AND THE RULES

In an early study of management now considered a classic (Mintzberg, 1973), the word "management" implied that a man filled the role. Leadership in health care was no different. Few women headed health care organizations until recently, and even men in nursing experience the same cultural environment and expectations as female nurses.

Gender Stereotypes

Helgesen and Johnson (2010) report that men and women view the world differently. Women, they assert, observe the world broadly, attending to people as well as tasks; men focus mainly on the job at hand. Table 2-2 lists differences in common stereotypes of men and women.

How do we reconcile the world of business, where men's attention to action fits the rules, with women's natural tendency toward inclusiveness and sharing? Helgesen and Johnson (2010) assert that women's style of leadership is just what the world of business needs.

What do women need to learn about work that they might not have learned growing up female? Table 2-3 illustrates some of the differences between traditional feminine and masculine expectations from work. Women, generally, have viewed work as an environment conducive to relationships. They want to be liked, to be inclusive, and to develop friendships, and they expect others to recognize their good work.

Men view work as goal-directed and success-oriented. They want to win the game, and they target their actions accordingly, developing relationships with people who can help them get ahead and making certain that others know what they've accomplished.

Today, these differences have blurred somewhat, and both men and women in nursing may have a variety of expectations from work. In addition, a recent study of male and female nurses' professional values reveals few differences between them (Alfred, Yarbrough, Martin & Garcia, 2011).

TABLE 2-2 Traditional Male and Female Stereotypes

Male Stereotype	Female Stereotype
Analytical	Intuitive
Linear-thinking	Dimensional-thinking
Aggressive	Deferential
Unfeeling	Empathetic
Competitive	Cooperative

TABLE 2-3 Traditional Feminine and Masculine Expectations from Work*

Masculine Expectations	Feminine Expectations
To be successful	To be liked
To make colleagues	To make friends
Just want to win	Everyone to win
Include those who can help me	To be included
Get money and other perks	Get praise and recognition
Expect to toot my own horn	Expect others to recognize my worth
To use this job to land a better one	To do my job well
Build relationships to help my career	Share my problems with others
Willing to take risks	To avoid risks

*These statements are generalities; both men and women exhibit a range of traits from both columns.

Belief that heterogeneity takes advantage of the talents and the skills of all regardless of individuals' gender, race, ethnicity, or disability undergirds all the civil rights' legislation of the last several decades. This is the same argument women used to gain access to professions and jobs that men held. Nursing, unfortunately, has a history of denying men equal opportunity.

Men in Nursing

As a man entering nursing in the mid-20th century, Luther Christman reports experiencing numerous examples of discrimination then and throughout his career (Christman, 2000). Furthermore, Christman says that organized nursing vigorously opposed efforts to recruit men to nursing. He suggests that if concerted efforts to recruit men had been made in the past, today's nursing shortage might never exist. In spite of opposition, Christman went on to be dean of the nursing schools at Vanderbilt University and Rush University and to serve in many high-level leadership positions in nursing and health care. More recently, male nurses have reported similar prejudices (Ramiccio, 2010).

Of the population of more than 3 million nurses in the United States, only 6 percent were men in 1990, although positive changes suggest the ratio is improving. The proportion of men to women has risen to 10 percent (U.S. Department of Health & Human Services, 2010).

In addition, a national ad campaign designed to recruit men asks, "Are You Man Enough to Be a Nurse?" It specifically targets the stereotype that nursing is only for females and that men aren't caring enough to be nurses (Ramiccio, 2010).

How Technology Changed the Workplace

Computerization has not only revolutionized work and personal life, but has also rendered it gender-neutral. In the past, men and women used different tools at work. Men operated heavy equipment, such as manufacturing or farm machinery, while women managed the home—handling cooking utensils and irons, for example—or worked in an office, using typewriters. The earliest nurses managed patients with little more than caring attitudes.

Today, men and women use the same tool—the computer. It may sit on a desk, travel in a laptop or notebook, or ride in a pocket as a smart phone. Regardless its structure or physical location, it connects to the world through cables and satellites. Whether accessing data, sending a message, or disseminating a report, the correspondent's gender is not a factor. The quality of the work matters; gender not at all (Helgesen & Johnson, 2010).

Although challenges to both men and women remain, technology continues to evolve, changing forever the ways people keep informed and interact. Information (accurate or inaccurate) is disseminated with lightening speed; social media connects diverse populations; and cell phones capture real-time events, broadcasting images instantaneously.

Technology has shrunk the world, and personal privacy is a myth. Surveillance cameras, cell phones, and magnetic entry cards track movements and activities. Worldwide business is the norm. Books, for that matter, can be accessed online and sold anywhere in the world.

HOW ORGANIZATIONS FUNCTION

Organizations, like individuals, value success. That may mean making money, positioning the organization to take advantage of future opportunities, generating community goodwill, or all of the above.

Most organizations today operate within the rules. They are hierarchical, with an identified chain of command that determines reporting relationships between positions. For example, the chief nurse reports to the hospital administrator, who is in turn responsible to the board of directors. The administrator expects the chief nurse to keep her informed about the nursing staff and to inform the nursing staff about hospital policies and decisions. Theoretically, this arrangement is expected to keep the organization functioning.

Staff versus Line Positions

Do you know the difference between a staff position and a line position? In most organizations, you know who your boss is. You also know whom you supervise, if you do. Therein lies the difference.

The line position carries with it influence and power, and the staff position has neither, per se, although some people in staff positions are able to accumulate influence. The experienced ward clerk is an example.

People in line positions have clout. They control budgets and can hire and fire staff. They are the power brokers of the organizations. Sometimes people who don't know the rules think they have power because they do important work and have an impressive title (titles are cheap). Their work may be very important to the success of the organization, but without clout, their influence is limited.

Responsibility without Authority

Responsibility and authority are often assumed to coexist. They do not, although they go together. If a person is given responsibility to do a task but lacks the authority to complete it, the job goes undone. This is a common situation in the workplace if managers fail to understand that authority must accompany responsibility to achieve a successful outcome.

Status Symbols

"Who needs them?" you might think. Doing good work speaks for itself. Wrong. Status symbols tell who's winning the game. Your status is partly determined by the status of the person to whom you report and how close that person is to the top. Doctors' parking areas and private dining room indicate the status of physicians in the hospital. The corner office does the same in the hierarchy of hospital administration or universities. Every item that an employee receives is counted, from office furniture to the square feet of space allotted.

Women, Evans (2000) asserts, tend to dismiss the value of status symbols, thinking they are saving the organization money and space if they don't ask for them even if men in similar positions have them. "I can do good work anywhere," one newly appointed chief nurse said after seeing her cramped office and used furniture. She is probably right, but there are other considerations. What image of nursing is she portraying when the other administrators demanded and received larger offices and new furniture?

Personal attire is also a status symbol. Do you remember your first nursing uniform? Whether it was a scrub suit or a white dress, your outfit symbolized your newly acquired status as a nurse. A lab coat over street clothes conveys a different image than a rumpled scrub suit. (You will learn more about clothing and image in Chapter 4.)

Many other items serve as status symbols. Where you live, with whom you socialize, and what your spouse does for a living are examples. Most of these you don't control—nor do you want to. Regardless, you should be aware of them.

> The nurse administrator of a large university medical center was driving to a meeting in a nearby city. Because her own car was in the shop for service, she borrowed a car from the fleet maintained by the university. The car was several years old and dented in a number of places. When she returned from the meeting in the late afternoon, she passed her secretary walking to the parking lot with a staff member from another department. "You'd think she could afford a better car," the staff member told her secretary. Remember this when you land that top-level job!

Leadership, Management, and Influence

Although leadership is taught in school and encouraged throughout a nurse's career, many individual nurses are unaware of their potential to promote their goals and affect health care beyond their immediate environment (e.g., individual patients, one unit, a clinic). Often, they are under the mistaken impression that leadership is fine for those nurses destined for management positions and that there is little need for practicing clinicians to develop these skills. In fact, many believe that leadership is an inborn characteristic that is incongruent with a nurse's commitment to care for patients. In reality, however, the skills to influence are available to anyone and can be taught, learned, and used to create a better future for health and nursing. (See Sullivan [2013] for help in enhancing your leadership and management skills.)

Assessing the Organizational Culture

Organizational culture refers to the norms and traditions that are maintained in the organization over time (Sullivan, 2013). Every organization has a culture unique to it. The organization's culture has evolved over the years, just as ethnic cultures have developed certain norms and traditions. Language, dress, rules, rituals, and customs are known but are not reported anywhere. The organizational culture can be positive and further the organization's goals as well as support individuals within the organization. Conversely, the organizational culture can be stifling or bureaucratic or can reward power grabbers, for example.

Culture is maintained regardless of the individuals in it. Have you even noticed that even when a troublemaker leaves, someone else takes on that person's role? That is the organizational culture operating. The norm has been set, and seldom does it change significantly unless radical forces, from outside the organization or inside it, alter it.

One force for change can be new administrative personnel. A determined, savvy leader can effect a culture change. In fact, sometimes administrators are hired to "clean up the place"—an order that, if carried out, expends a huge amount of the administrator's power capital and often leads to the administrator leaving the organization after the changes are implemented.

The change may or may not remain after the administrator is gone; whether it does depends on many other factors, including who replaces the administrator. One reason for the popularity of consultants for work redesign and organizational restructuring is that outside consultants can come in, make their recommendations, and leave. The administrators responsible for making the changes are one step removed from the changes.

Subcultures also exist in organizations, and they too have norms and traditions. Nursing, for example, forms a subculture in health care organizations. So do physicians and the housekeeping and maintenance staff. Each subculture has its own expectations for members, its own jargon, and its implied understandings.

At times, these subcultures can clash. If male values predominate, such a hierarchical, bureaucratic system will fail to incorporate the networking and community building more often promoted by women (Morgan, 2007).

Or the subcultures may complement each other. Morgan (2007) suggests that the trend is toward more inclusive, participative organizational structures that incorporate gender, ethnic, and professional differences.

Regardless of the formal structure and the informal working relationships that predominate in the work setting, everyone must conform—at least in some degree—to the organizational culture and subculture's norms.

HOW WORK DIFFERS FROM SOCIAL SETTINGS

It's not personal; it's business. Here's how to recognize the difference between work and social life: if anyone else in your same position would receive the same treatment, then it's business. If a patient's father yells at you because he thinks you're not doing enough for his son, it's business. If the hospital administrator complains that you're racking up too much overtime, it's business. If you have to fire someone because of poor performance or budget cuts, it's business. In all of these cases, it's not personal.

One of the best lessons you can learn is that you are not your job, and whatever happens to you on the job is not personal.

Health care is a business, whether we like it or not. Even nonprofit enterprises are businesses. They only differ from for-profit organizations in the way they use funds that exceed costs; nonprofits reinvest them in the organization and for-profit organizations pay revenues above expenses to their stockholders.

Work is about success; social life is about pleasure and approval. Work is not a popularity contest and is not meant to provide you with friends (although you might become friends with people you meet through work). You can cancel or miss a social function or even drop out of a social group if you don't like the people, don't agree with their goals or activities, or don't like where they meet or their hours. The repercussions, per se, will not affect your income or success.

Not so with work. We are expected to show up, suited up and ready to work at an assigned time and place. In return we receive pay and—hopefully—recognition and opportunity for advancement if we want.

Knowing When to Break, Bend, or Ignore the Rules

Rules are not meant to be followed without question, and there are times when you should break them, bend them a bit, or ignore them completely. You must know, however, when, where, and how to violate them. You can decide to defy the rules if you think the potential benefits will outweigh any repercussions that you are willing to accept. Usually, these are minor issues for management but important to you, especially if you think the long-term gain is worth it. People who are effective change makers often say they'd rather beg forgiveness than ask permission.

> A nurse faculty member was offered a job by the dean, who asked the faculty member to become her assistant. The faculty member was interested in administration and thought this would be a good opportunity to learn about becoming an administrator. She would work with the dean, represent her within the university and at local organizations at times; in short, she would learn a tremendous amount about becoming an administrator. It sounded like just what the faculty member wanted.
>
> Then the dean said her title would be "assistant to the dean." The faculty member asked if anyone would report to her. The answer was no. The faculty member asked if she would handle any budgets. Again the answer was no. Nor would the faculty member hire anyone. The dean assured her, though, that she would be involved in all those activities at the dean's side.
>
> The faculty member declined the position, though she mentioned that she would accept it with the title of assistant dean. She knew that assistant dean would be a more impressive title on her résumé than assistant to the dean. Even though the job was still not a line position, the faculty member knew she would learn a great deal from this successful dean who could also serve as her mentor.
>
> The dean agreed to the title of assistant dean, and the faculty member's experience helped her eventually to become a dean herself. She knew the rules and knew when it was to her advantage to break them.

You can evaluate the pros and cons of moving ahead with your goals and decide whether it is worth it. Maybe the outcome is so good that you can take a chance. Just don't do it too often.

Some rules are more absolute than others. Here are some:

Never bad-mouth your boss.

Never avoid paying a debt.

Never sabotage the team.

Never, never lie.

WHY NURSING DOESN'T FIT THE RULES

Nursing doesn't fit easily into the rules for many reasons. One, of course, is that we're in a predominantly female profession, for all the reasons described in previous pages. The nature of nursing work also doesn't fit the rules. Nursing is inherently a feel-good profession. For us, to care for others, to help them manage their illnesses and their treatments, and to know that we are caring for people when they are most vulnerable is the reward of being in this satisfying profession.

Nursing's Rules

What are some of nursing's rules? Do you agree that the following are the unwritten rules in nursing?

No one nurse is more important than another.

Everyone should stay at the same level.

Don't brag.

Give credit to others.

Include everyone.

When you say, "The patient learned . . ." instead of "I taught her . . ." or "Any nurse would do it" when you did it, and the common favorite, "You'll have to ask the doctor," you may fit the nursing culture, but your statements do little to enlighten anyone about nursing's role in health care.

Can you think of some more unwritten rules? Are these rules prevalent in your organization?

Being a Victim

How many times have you heard nurses complain about their jobs? Too often to count? And to whom do they complain? Other nurses! Complaining to each other does little to change what is wrong, whether it's our hours, a difficult patient, or an argument with a physician.

Marie Manthey, founder of the consulting firm Creative Nursing Management, says, "Deliver the mail to the right address." When we talk about our problems to people who are not involved and unlikely to be able to help, we do two things: first, we get it off our chest. We feel better and can go on about our work until something else happens. Then we're back to the same place, tell our friends again, and the cycle continues. No real change occurs.

Do you see how change cannot occur if we don't deliver our message to the right person? Remember the student who was afraid to apply to graduate school because he might not be accepted? The same is true in delivering your message, regardless of whether we were successful in getting what we wanted. If you don't give it to the right person, change cannot occur.

Even in professional organizations, nurses often are reluctant to develop relationships with powerful leaders outside of nursing who could further our goals. One nurse leader had an opportunity to honor a person who had contributed to her career. Most of her predecessors had honored other nurses, but this nurse did not. She carefully chose a physician who had mentored her executive career and who was well-known in medical and health care circles. What he learned about nurses' contributions to health care was only reinforced when he attended the event where he was honored. How he might use this information in the future, no one knew—and would maybe never find out. What we all know is that his view of nursing leadership was enhanced; that could do no harm.

Sometimes it seems easier to remain a victim. Our colleagues agree with us, making us feel included. Nothing is as bad when it's shared. Some problems, mostly personal ones, can be shared with close friends. Work life is not the same as your personal life, and the goal of solving a problem is to address the source. Otherwise, the problem is just perpetuated.

MAKING THE RULES WORK FOR YOU

We have two options: follow the rules and win, or ignore them and complain. The sports and military analogies are offensive to some nurses. So be it. This is the real world of work. If we want to play in it, we must follow the rules.

How can you use the rules to further your goals and nursing's agenda? Here are some ideas:

Speak up for yourself, your patients, your profession.

Don't assume responsibility without authority.

Don't do the dirty work alone.

Accept the risk.

Don't be a victim.

Learn when to break, bend, or ignore the rules. Decide when you are willing to beg for forgiveness rather than ask permission.

Caring for Ourselves

As nurses, we get fulfillment from caring for others. We are inclined to dismiss the importance of caring for ourselves. We must come to realize that we can care for ourselves with the same attention we give our patients. (See Chapter 14 for more on how to care for yourself.)

We deserve to be enthusiastic about the work we do and to find satisfaction in it at the same time. We have a right to be rewarded for our endeavors.

Melodie Chenevert has promoted the rights of nurses throughout her speaking and writing career. She asserts that women—and, we would add, men—in the health professions have the ten basic rights shown in Table 2-4.

How Nurses Can Succeed

Ultimately, nurses' abilities to establish and maintain relationships can enable us to achieve greater success as long as we do not let relationships supersede our work goals. It's all in how we learn to use these skills in various areas of our work and lives. This book discusses how you can build on the relationship skills you already have as a nurse to become the influential person you can be.

Imagine that every nurse working today, this very minute, was excited and satisfied in his or her job. What a transformation our health care system would see!

TABLE 2-4 Ten Basic Rights for Men and Women in Nursing

1. You have the right to be treated with respect.
2. You have the right to a reasonable workload.
3. You have the right to an equitable wage.
4. You have the right to determine your own priorities.
5. You have the right to ask for what you want.
6. You have the right to refuse without making excuses or feeling guilty.
7. You have the right to make mistakes and be responsible for them.
8. You have the right to give and receive information as a professional.
9. You have the right to act in the best interest of the patient.
10. You have the right to be human.

Adapted from Chenevert, M. (1993). *STAT: Special techniques in assertiveness training for women in the health professions.* St. Louis: Mosby. Used with permission.

What You Know Now

You have learned about the game of work, the game board (i.e., the organizational structure), and the rules. You know some characteristics of organizations and how to assess your organization's culture. You know now that your work life and your social life are different. You've learned some gender differences in how men and women approach work and why nursing doesn't fit naturally into the rules. You also are able to assess when you might bend, break, or ignore the rules. Now you are ready to make the rules work for you.

Remember, life is an adventure. Enjoy it!

Tools for Using the Rules

1. Use every opportunity to observe the rules in action.
2. Incorporate the rules into the relationship skills you already have.
3. Review the Ten Basic Rights for Men and Women in Nursing (Table 2-4). Memorize them if you can.
4. Make a commitment to take care of yourself.

Learning Activities

1. Make two lists. Name one list "What I owe." In a few words, jot down as many recent instances as you can remember when you asked someone for advice, help, information, or a favor. Opposite each favor, put the person's name who helped you.

   Now make another list. Title this one "What others owe me." Jot down instances when someone else asked you for help and put their names beside the event.

   Look at both lists. Did you help others more than they helped you? Evaluate the magnitude of each favor. Working a holiday for you is greater than picking up supplies on the way back from lunch, for example. Using a scale of 1 to 5 (5 being the most helpful), calculate what you owe each person and what others owe you.

Wait for when you need something from someone who owes you. Remind the person about what you did and ask for what you want. Be tactful but direct. If the person agrees, mentally mark that debt paid. Pay attention to how you and others use this system.

2. Assess your organization's culture. What are the prevailing values? How do your values fit with the organization's?

   Now assess the values of the subculture of nursing in your organization. Does it fit with organization's culture? How could you help make it fit better?

   Decide if you can live with any differences. If not, think about exploring work at another organization.

3. Review the example earlier in this chapter of the nurse who didn't know whether she should support her mentor or not when the mentor was about to be fired. Decide what you would do and justify your answer.

   Ask several classmates or colleagues to do the same. Then compare answers. Here's a hint: the mentor may go on to bigger and better positions.

References

Alfred, D., Yarbrough, S., Martin, P., & Garcia, C. (2011). Gender and professional values: A closer look. *Nursing Management, 42*(1), 34–36.

Baber, A., & Waymon, L. (2007). *Make your contacts count* (2nd ed.). New York: American Management Association.

Chenevert, M. (1993). *STAT: Special techniques in assertiveness training for women in the health professions.* St. Louis: Mosby.

Christman, L. (2000). Letter to the editor. *Journal of Professional Nursing, 17*(1), 3.

Evans, G. (2000). *Play like a man, win like a woman: What men know about success that women need to learn.* New York: Broadway Books.

Evans, G. (2003). *She wins, you win.* New York: Gotham Books.

Grossman, S. C. (2007). *Mentoring in nursing: A dynamic and collaborative process.* New York: Springer Publishing.

Helgesen, S., & Johnson, J. (2010). *The female vision: Women's real power at work.* San Francisco: Berrett-Koehler Publications.

McDowell, J. B., Williams, R. L., Kautz, D. D., Madden, P., Heilig, A., & Thompson, A. (2010). Shared governance: 10 years later. *Nursing Management, 41*(7), 33–37.

Melia, J. (1986). *Breaking into the boardroom: What every woman needs to know when talent and hard work aren't enough.** New York: St. Martin's Press.

Mintzberg, H. (1973). *The nature of managerial work.* New York: Harper & Row.

Morgan, G. (2007). *Images of organization.* Thousand Oaks, CA: Sage Publications.

Ramiccio, M. (April 8, 2010). Nursing ad campaigns take on the male stereotype. Retrieved October 15, 2010, from http://www.OrlandoSentinel.com

Sullivan, E. J. (2013). *Effective leadership and management in nursing* (8th ed.). Upper Saddle River, NJ: Prentice Hall Health.

U.S. Department of Health & Human Services, Health Resources and Service Administration (2010). *National sample survey of registered nurses.* Retrieved October 15, 2010, from http://bhpr.hrsa.gov/healthworkforce/rnsurvey2008.html

*Sadly, this book is out of print.

Web Resources

Manthey, Mary. Weblog. http://mariesnursingsalon.wordpress.com

Sullivan, E. J. Men in nursing: The importance of gender diversity. *Journal of Professional Nursing*, 16(5). Retrieved April 15, 2011, from http://www.eleanorsullivan.com/pdf/men.pdf

Sullivan, E. J. Nursing and feminism: An uneasy alliance. *Journal of Professional Nursing, 18*(4). Retrieved April 15, 2011, from http://www.eleanorsullivan.com/pdf/feminism.pdf

Sullivan, E. J. Rules of the game. Retrieved April 15, 2011, from http://www.eleanorsullivan.com/pdf/The_Rules_of_the_Game.pdf

Winslow, L. Beating the game even when the game is flawed. Retrieved April 15, 2011, from http://ezinearticles.com/?Beating-the-Game-Even-When-the-Game-is-Flawed&id=326610

CASE STUDY

Learning the Rules

Because he had enjoyed caring for palliative care patients on a medical unit, Will was pleased when he was chosen for a position on the home hospice team. During orientation, Evan (his preceptor) taught him the hospice team's routines and protocols.

Although the work with patients was satisfying, Will didn't feel like part of the team. The congenial group of nurses worked together, talking frequently, sharing weekend call, and offering clinical advice to each other. Will planned to work on this team for a long time to come, and he needed to find a way to fit in with the team better.

Deciding that Evan might be able to help, Will invited him to lunch and explained his problem. "Can you help me?" he asked Evan.

"It's not personal," Evan explained. "We've all worked together for several years, and I guess we're comfortable with each other."

"So what do you suggest?"

"How about we meet every third Wednesday for lunch," Evan offered. "I can catch you up so you stay in the loop."

"That'd be great. Thanks. And I'll post my cell number on the team bulletin board so if people need to trade weekend call, they'd be comfortable asking me."

"Good idea. Say, you've had experience with IV pumps, haven't you?"

"Yes. Even the latest ones."

"Most of us aren't that familiar with them, and that's a problem when a patient with a pump's admitted to our hospice care group."

Will finished Evan's idea. "I could volunteer to take care of that patient."

"Don't worry, Will," Evan assured him. "You'll soon be one of us."

Will's colleagues responded to his offers, and it wasn't long before Will felt connected to the team and comfortable in his job.

3

Understanding and Using Your Power

We have, I fear, confused power with greatness.

STEWART UDALL DARTMOUTH COLLEGE, 1965

In this chapter, you will learn:

- What power is
- How to use power appropriately
- How power can be undermined or misused
- What happens when power is not used appropriately
- How to handle power plays

POWER DEFINED

Power is the potential ability to influence (Hersey, Blanchard, & Johnson, 2007). Power enables you to make choices, create order, mobilize resources, bring about change, and be effective in your work and your life. Power differs from influence in that power describes the capacity to be influential and influence itself is the use of that power. These are minor but important distinctions because often power is not used to influence. This book exists to help nurses recognize and use their power.

Authority is sometimes confused with power. Authority is based on one's position, usually a formal role in an organization, such as the CEO of a hospital or the president of the American Nurses Association. When the person leaves the position, the authority that went with the position disappears. Power, however, may be retained or even enhanced depending on the person's reputation and influence.

A balance of power is preferred so that one person or group is prevented from assuming control of the larger entity. The three branches of the federal government are an example. An organization (e.g., university, hospital, professional association) is governed by a board of directors for the same reason. Absolute power exists only in a dictatorship. Everyone else answers to someone. Even the president of the United States answers to the electorate and must cooperate with Congress, and the president's power can be nullified by rulings from the U.S. Supreme Court.

Power is involved in every human encounter, regardless of whether you recognize it. Power can be symmetrical when two parties have equal and reciprocal power, or it may be asymmetrical with one person or group holding more control than another (Mason, Leavitt, & Chaffee, 2011). Power can be exclusive to one party or shared among many people or groups.

Principle-centered power is a model congruent with nursing's values. It is based on respect, honor, loyalty, and commitment. Originally conceived by Stephen Covey (1990), today the model is increasingly used by leaders in many fields (Ikeda, 2009). Power sharing evolves naturally when power is centered on one's values and principles. In fact, the notion that power is something to be shared seems to contradict the usual belief that power is something to be amassed, protected, and used for one's own purposes.

Nurses can accept power as positive and necessary, but they do not need to grab power for its own sake. This is a difficult distinction that individuals continue to struggle with long after they have risen to positions of influence. (See the section "Inappropriate Use of Power" later in this chapter.)

For the Novice Nurse

What power do I have, you ask? New to the profession and the health care setting, you find that everyone has power except you. But that's not so. In this chapter, you'll learn how to make the most of the power of your work, your words, and your influence. More important, you'll learn how to avoid undermining yourself or failing to use your power. Power, you ask again?

You have more than you think.

TYPES OF POWER

Power attached to a formal position is easily recognized (Morgan, 2007). The dean of a school of nursing has power, for instance. Some people, however, seem to have power without such a visible sign. The ward clerk on a hospital unit does not have an administrative role, but the clerk has power in the unit—as anyone who has ever worked in a hospital knows. How? With *information*, one source of power. (See Table 3-1 for the types of power.)

TABLE 3-1 Types of Power

Type	Definition
Position	Associated with one's role in the organization
Information	Based on individual's access to valuable information
Expert	Individual has valuable and unique expertise
Personal	Person is respected for reputation, credibility
Connection	Based on formal and informal links to influential people
Perceived	Individual has reputation for power

Still others have power because they are *experts*. Your IT tech has power when your computer goes down. Some people have power because they are respected, which is one form of *personal* power. Religious leaders wield that kind of power. Still others have power because of the people they know. The neighbor of a state legislator has power because the neighbor may be able to lobby the legislator for funding for your school of nursing, for example. This type is known as *connection* power.

Someone with power has the ability to reward or punish other people, organizations, businesses, or causes. Or they are perceived to be able to do so. How does that happen? If people believe that a person or group has power, known as *perceived* power, the effect is the same regardless of how much power they actually hold over you. The IRS, your boss, and your instructor in college are examples. Some actually have power but may not have to use it because you believe they can.

The Surgeon General of the United States has no actual authority, but he or she wields power because people perceive that the person holding the office has power. Such a position is known as a "bully pulpit." This person's words alone can be influential. Several decades ago, Surgeon General C. Everett Koop reported the dangers of smoking, resulting in efforts that continue successfully today to reduce smoking.

Nurses have power in several of these areas. Those who hold leadership positions have power. Nurses have expert power, informational power, connection power (who else can call a physician in the middle of the night?), relationship power, and personal power.

So why don't they use it? Is it possible that nurses don't recognize the power that they have? Do they think others have more power?

HOW TO USE YOUR POWER

Using Power Correctly

Every use of power is embedded in interactions with others and enhances or diminishes the relationship. The rules for using power are shown in Table 3-2. A general rule is to use the least amount of power to produce the

TABLE 3-2 Rules for Using Power

1. Use the least amount of power you can to be effective in your interactions with others.
2. Use power appropriate to the situation.
3. Learn when not to use power.
4. Focus on the problem, not the person.
5. Make polite requests, never arrogant demands.
6. Use coercion only when other methods don't work.
7. Keep informed to retain your credibility when using your expert power.
8. Understand that you may owe a return favor when you use your connection power.

results you want (e.g., "Don't use a hammer to swat a fly."). For example, say you want a nursing assistant to pass meal trays. You can ask (using minimal power), demand/insist (more powerful than a simple request), or threaten consequences (e.g., disciplinary action) if the trays are not delivered in a timely manner.

Using the least amount of power is especially important if you have an ongoing relationship with the person. People have long memories, and an angry confrontation will be remembered by the person involved and anyone who observed it. Others, too, will hear about the altercation. You are building a reputation. Each encounter sets the stage for future ones with that person and his or her friends, colleagues, and coworkers. You may have won that battle but may ultimately lose the war.

Power should also be appropriate to the situation. Sometimes you need to use the most power you have—when a patient codes, for example. When a direct order is needed is not the time to make a request.

On the other hand, certain circumstances can be resolved without any use of power. For instance, a nurse manager observing two employees quarreling about a minor issue can step in and try to resolve the issue or wait to see if the two people can settle their differences. The manager may not need to use his positional power at all.

Other rules for using power include retaining a focus on the problem without attacking the person and making polite requests rather than arrogant demands. Use coercion only when you've tried less powerful means without results. To maintain credibility when using your informational power, be sure to keep yourself informed. And remember, you may incur a debt when you use your connections with others to further your goals.

Increasing Your Power

Many people falsely believe that power is limited and that they cannot acquire more power. Several strategies can be used to increase your power in all areas of your life. Doing so is known as expanding your *power base*.

TABLE 3-3 Strategies to Increase Your Power Base

1. Increase your level of involvement in the organization.
2. Do your job with efficiency and effectiveness. Take on extra responsibilities as you are able.
3. Learn all you can about the organization and the people in it.
4. Be visible in the organization.
5. Ask for help and advice.
6. Associate with the power players as appropriate.
7. Network within the organization and in as many other places as you can.
8. Share your power with others; it will come back twofold.
9. Continue to develop yourself and your skills.

The power of people you know and the relationships you have with them constitute your power base, which explains why people often try to get to know those in power positions whose attractiveness has little to do with them personally and everything to do with their position. This attempt is not wrong; it is part of the game. Remember, though, that it's business, and when one is no longer in power, the relationship may end.

A number of strategies can be used to increase your power base. Table 3-3 lists some of them. These strategies can be used in your workplace, professional associations, and community or religious organizations.

Undermining Your Power

WHINING. The best way to undermine your power is by whining. Complaining about everything that makes your life difficult—such as the weather, traffic, your spouse, your boss, or your coworkers—is whining. Whining marks you as a pathetic loser in the real world of work. Today's busy hospital or clinic needs all the attention, energy, and concentration of every employee. The workplace is no place for whining.

EXCUSES. Excuses are a close second to whining and illustrate some of the reasons people give for whining. A reason, of course, is not an excuse; it is just a reason, that is, a problem to be solved or a situation to be corrected. "I didn't have time" and "No one would help me" are excuses heard every day in a workplace somewhere.

These statements may be true, but they are not reasons to be defeated. Solving problems by exploring alternative solutions is what marks the winner, not the loser. Taking a chance is always risky. (Remember what you learned in Chapters 1 and 2 about risk.) If you don't get the results you want, you need another strategy, not an excuse. No amount of discussion about all the ways you tried will solve the problem. Results-oriented people understand that trying something matters not at all; only the outcome is important.

KILLER PHRASES. Some excuses qualify as killer phrases. That is, they effectively shut down communication and engender feelings of defeat and resignation. You have heard all of these.

"She'll get mad."

"They'll think I'm showing off."

"It'll cost too much."

"We tried that before."

"Administration won't go for it."

Whether you're suggesting an idea to address a patient's problem or proposing a new clinic service, you can be discouraged if you hear any of these reactions. But there are ways to handle them. Keep calm and let the person talk. If someone brings up something you hadn't thought of, admit that you need more information and seek the group's help. Ask questions, take notes, and think about how you can answer arguments without driving others into an entrenched position where they erect mental barriers to the discussion, resulting in a "bunker mentality." If this happens, you may need to postpone the discussion and use the time to find solutions to your opponents' arguments.

No matter how well prepared you are or how much you've countered every argument, everything you try won't always work. That's the risk of taking chances. It's also the opportunity for success.

EMOTIONAL REACTIONS. Reacting emotionally is self-defeating. Becoming angry, crying, sulking, or refusing to talk (e.g., "never mind," "it's not important") undermines your power at that moment and in the future. If you feel like you cannot control your emotions, try to do so until you can excuse yourself and take time to regain your composure. Remind yourself that it's not personal; it's just business.

REFUSING TO ADMIT MISTAKES. Everyone makes mistakes, even influential people. Sometimes these are minor errors; other times they may be more serious, involving patient safety. It is important to understand the difference in order to respond accordingly.

The seriousness is determined by the consequences. Being a few minutes late to work is minor; failing to give a patient medication is serious. Sometimes, though, people don't discriminate between the two.

Guilt, shame, and fear are normal reactions to making a mistake. So are making excuses and blaming others. A better way—the way those with influence use—is to admit your mistake, offer to fix it, and move on. A mistake is just a mistake. No more, no less.

If the system needs changing (e.g., automatic prompts when incompatible medications are ordered), this is a perfect time to suggest a way to fix it. Regardless of whether changes occur, you have learned something you might not have known (e.g., don't rely on the pharmacy to check for compatibility of meds).

Mistakes are opportunities for learning your weaknesses. They call attention to problems you need to address. You undermine your power when you fail to admit mistakes, correct what you can, and let it go. Don't use excuses in lieu of results. Take responsibility for what is entrusted to you.

When You Don't Use Your Power

When you fail to use the power you have by virtue of your position, your expertise, or your access to information, you miss opportunities for yourself, your patients, and your profession. You are likely to appear indecisive and to be perceived as less able than you are. Your credibility is diminished, thereby reducing your effectiveness in the future. Your opinion is likely to be dismissed; in fact, you may be overlooked in many situations.

> The chief nurse for a large, metropolitan hospital reported that salary decisions for nurses had already been made by an administrative group by the time she heard about it. Her response to the problem was a shrug and a comment that "it was already done."

This situation illustrates an important aspect of power. Although the supply is unlimited, there seems to be a critical mass in any organization or group. When the critical mass is reached (that is, a group seems to hold all the power), others are left out. The chief of nursing in the example scenario was not in the power group. Unless something changed in the organization, such as a restructuring of the administrative group, this nurse was unlikely to obtain more power. She must decide if she is willing to stay with the organization and accept her power limits, try to acquire more power by working with one or two key influential people, or leave the organization. It is seldom that any of us have all the power we need—much less want—but knowing where, when, and how we have power enables us to make informed decisions about our work and our future.

Inappropriate Use of Power

Power, appropriately used, can be a force to help you achieve your goals. Power can also be used inappropriately. Power can be underused, misused, or overused.

Power that is not used when it is needed (i.e., underused) results in a loss of credibility and a perception of incompetence. The person is perceived to lack concern for the group and to be out of touch with the situation.

If someone continually makes poor decisions or fails to make decisions, power is lost. When your boss ignores inadequate performance and gives everyone equal rewards (praise or monetary rewards), her power base is eroded. She is under using her power.

Power is misused when a person fails to match the power to the situation. Underuse is one example; overuse is another. You probably can remember a time when someone overreacted to a situation, especially if that person was in a power position, such as a teacher or supervisor.

Overuse of power sows fear and hostility in others. It stifles creativity and problem solving. The person who overuses power tends to be avoided as much as possible, and information is selectively filtered to avoid an angry response. Lack of trust results; thus, the person's ability to meet goals is diminished. Remember to use the least amount of power necessary to achieve your results and to use that power appropriately and judiciously.

Power must fit the organization, the situation, and the maturity and competence of those involved. A general rule is: the more decentralized the organization, the more important the maturity and competence of the people closest to the action (e.g., patient care). Also, the relative importance of the situation bears on the power used. In an emergency, it is appropriate to demand action. During a code, for example, no one expects to be treated gently. On the other hand, a request to go to lunch early deserves courtesy even if you have the power to just tell others. Remember, you're building a relationship, not just engaging in a one-time interaction.

HOW TO HANDLE POWER PLAYS

Power plays are manipulative attempts to undermine or demolish others. Even savvy players are sometimes thrown by these. Typical power plays include:

"Let's be fair."

"Can you prove that?"

"It's either this or that; which is it? Take your pick."

"But you said . . . and now you say. . . ."

Such statements engender feelings of insecurity, incompetence, confusion, embarrassment, and anger. You do not need to respond directly in these situations; rather, you can simply restate your initial point in a firm manner. Keep your expression neutral, ignore accusations, and restate your position, if appropriate. If you refuse to respond to such thinly veiled attacks, your opponent is unable to intimidate and manipulate you.

Similar to the effect of other interactions, both opponents and others will soon recognize that you are a savvy player, and these attempts to discredit you should diminish in time. (Bullying is a special case of intimidation that is discussed in Chapter 10.)

What You Know Now

You have learned that power describes the potential to influence, so you can be effective in your work and your life. You know about the different types of power and that nurses may not realize the power they have. You have learned how to use power correctly and how to increase your power base. You also know how power can be used inappropriately. You know how you can undermine your own power and what happens when you don't use the power you have. Finally, you have learned how to handle power plays. You know that power is a positive force in your game arsenal.

Ready to use your power appropriately? Go!

Tools for Power

1. Learn the rules for using power and put them into practice.
2. Increase your power base by using the strategies suggested.
3. Remember situations in which you failed to use your power. Try to use your power in similar circumstances in the future.
4. Guard against undermining your power or using power inappropriately.

Learning Activities

1. Pick three people you encounter frequently who are in positions of power, such as your instructor, a supervisor, or a community leader. Observe their use of power in at least three situations. Ask the following questions:
   a. Did they use their power? If not, can you identify why?
   b. If they used their power, what type was it? Did they use their power correctly?
   c. Did you observe any attempts to intimidate them? If so, how did they handle them?
   Share your experiences with classmates or colleagues.
2. Select an organization where you would like to increase your power. You may use your workplace, school, or professional or community organization. Rate yourself on a scale from 1 (poor) to 5 (excellent) as follows:
   ________ Level of involvement
   ________ Efficiency and effectiveness
   ________ Acceptance of extra responsibilities
   ________ Knowledge about the organization
   ________ Visibility
   ________ Asking for help and advice
   ________ Associating with power players
   ________ Networking
   ________ Sharing power
   ________ Developing yourself
   Think about how you can increase your power using the strategies shown in Table 3-3.
3. Role-play various scenarios, using information in this chapter, that demonstrate increasing your power, using power inappropriately, and undermining your power. You can use one partner, or three people can participate with one person as the observer. Create typical situations to challenge each other.

References

Covey, S. R. (1991). *Principle-centered leadership*. New York: Simon & Schuster.

Hersey, P., Blanchard, K. H., & Johnson, D. (2007). *Management of organizational behavior: Utilizing human resources* (9th ed.). Englewood Cliffs, NJ: Prentice Hall.

Ikeda, J. (2009). Principle centered power. Retrieved April 12, 2011, from http://www.leadwithhonor.com/blog/2009/03/26/principle-centered-power/

Mason, D. J., Leavitt, J. K., & Chaffee, M. W. (2011). *Policy and politics in nursing and health care* (6th ed.). Philadelphia: W. B. Saunders.

Morgan, G. (2007). *Images of organization.* Thousand Oaks, CA: Sage Publications.

Web Resources

Ponte, P. R., Glazer, G., Dann, E., McCollum, K., Gross, A., Tyrrell, R., et al. (2007). The power of professional nursing practice: An essential element of patient and family centered care. *The Online Journal of Issues in Nursing, 12*(1). Retrieved April 15, 2011, from http://www.medscape.com/viewarticle/553405

Gilbert-Jamison, T. (2011). The power of professional presence: 20 basics for career advancement. Retrieved April 15, 2011, from http://ezinearticles.com/?The-Power-of-Professional-Presence—20-Basics-For-Career-Advancement&id=2185035

Print Resource

Marshall, S. (2000). *How to grow a backbone: 10 strategies for gaining power and influence at work.* Chicago: Contemporary Books.

CASE STUDY

Using Power

Because of her experience with orthopedic patients, Rosa was considered an expert by her peers and patients and often served as a preceptor to new nurses. In fact, last year she was nominated for a Preceptor of the Year award at her hospital.

After admitting her second patient of the night, Rosa spoke to her new nurse orientee, Linda. "Let's take a moment to regroup and plan care for the rest of the shift."

Rosa and Linda reviewed the vital signs of their patients from the 11:00 vital sign collection. They noted that Mr. Antiago in room 4918 had a blood pressure reading of 192/115.

"We need to check on him immediately," Rosa told Linda.

Upon entering his room, they noted Mr. Antiago grimacing in pain and perspiring. "I need pain medicine," he told them.

"Where does it hurt?" Rosa asked.

"Right here." He pointed to his surgery incision. Rosa retrieved the pain medicine ordered and administered it to Mr. Antiago. She then re-checked his blood pressure. It was 188/113.

"Are you having chest pains or trouble breathing?" Rosa asked him.

"No, but sometimes my pressure's high at home, and I take medicine for it."

"After giving pain meds and doing a recheck of the vital sign reading," Rosa explained to Linda, "our protocol is to call the physician if the reading's still abnormal."

"At home? At night?"

"Be prepared. Have all information with you and present it succinctly."

Linda looked doubtful.

Rosa paged Dr. Hollinghouse; when he returned the call, she explained Mr. Antiago's condition.

The doctor replied, "Administer Clonidine 0.1 mg for his high blood pressure by mouth and then recheck the blood pressure in one hour and call me back."

Rosa agreed. Her experience with Dr. Hollinghouse told that he appreciated her expertise and trusted her judgment.

One hour later, Rosa called Dr. Hollinghouse back. Mr. Antiago's blood pressure had improved. It read 132/84.

4

The Power of Image

Your expression is the most important thing you can wear.

SID ASCHER

In this chapter, you will learn:

- Why nursing's image matters
- How your image influences others
- How nurses are perceived
- What affects your image
- How to present a positive image

WHAT IS IMAGE?

Image reflects an unknown reality. Just as your image on a photograph is not you, your image is a reflection of you to others. What people know about you and what they can see are all they have to go on. They cannot see what you don't show them.

Image consists of the sum total of way you appear to others, including your appearance, words, behavior, and status (see Table 4-1). Who you are, what you do, your family, and what is known about your history (e.g., how much education you have and where you received it, your work history, your family's history) all contribute to the way others see you.

TABLE 4-1 Components of Image

Appearance
Weight, height, and body build
Clothing
Clean, pressed, repaired
Shoes clean without excessive wear
Jewelry, makeup, nail polish
Personal hygiene
Behavior
Posture
Gestures
Language
Choice of words
Manner of speaking
Grammar
Etiquette
Background
Family background
Educational history
Work history
Status
Living arrangements (neighborhood, suburb; house, apartment)
Car
Current position
Professional and volunteer work
Family situation (single, married, divorced, widowed; children, their ages, schools, accomplishments)

For the Novice Nurse

You have a rare opportunity to exhibit the image of nursing. Unlike your more experienced peers, you're starting fresh. How you appear, what you do, and how you do it affects your future and nursing's image. How's that for an onerous responsibility? But you're up to it, that's for certain.

You're a nurse!

Let's look at the components of your image: appearance, behavior, and surroundings. First, your appearance. Don't cringe. Nothing can be done to alter our basic body features, such as height and bone structure. Few of us want to alter our facial features, and only limited changes can be made to our hair. Also, most of us are restricted by what we can spend on clothing. So what can we change? Lots.

Aspects of your appearance that you can control include your weight, posture, cleanliness, and attire. Let's take weight, for example. Few people are actually satisfied with their weight, and many want to weigh less. Unfortunately, a person who is obviously obese projects a negative image in contemporary society. Obese people thus have less influence than their slender colleagues. Enough said. Nurses know about nutrition and can make their own decisions about habits that affect their weight and health.

Personal hygiene, clothing, body art, piercings, jewelry, and makeup contribute substantially to image and are often what we think of when considering image. Scrubs suits are common attire for nurses; they should be neat, clean, and pressed (LaSala & Nelson, 2005). A recent study found that patients perceived nurses in solid-color scrub suits and minimal body art as the most skilled, caring, and knowledgeable (Thomas et al., 2010). To convey an image of a competent professional ready to work, avoid oversized jewelry, bright nail polish, heavy makeup, or obvious tattoos.

Clothing matters even more when you are not wearing a uniform. Colorful prints may be appropriate for social events, but they distract from a professional image at work-related functions. Neutral colors such as tan, gray, black, brown, or navy allow attention to focus on you and not your clothing. In addition, black, navy, and red are power colors and can be worn to emphasize your expertise or to give you an edge in negotiations. Learn to distinguish between clothes that are cute or sexy and those that convey the professional image you want (LaSala & Nelson, 2005).

Posture can project an image of a confident and competent person or convey humility and subservience, in addition to many other attributes. Fortunately, posture is very amenable to correction, except for those with permanent disabilities. Posture reflects our opinion of ourselves. If you've ever watched a new nursing grad develop skills over time, you've probably seen this nurse switch from exhibiting a posture that suggests hesitancy and uncertainty to one that conveys pride and self-assurance. In addition to posture, your gestures, choice of language, and manner of speaking all affect your image.

Image is even affected by where you live and what car you drive. Don't you categorize people by attributes according to where their home is (e.g., upscale suburb or traditional neighborhood), whether they drive a SUV or a hybrid (or own a car at all), and their religion (if you know it)? We need to be able to put people into some group, at least initially, to have a sense of who they are until we get to know them better. Problems arise when we continue to have a limited perception of people without allowing for individual differences. At its worst, this categorization is known as stereotyping and has resulted in legislation to counter such discrimination.

Although you want to project a positive and professional image, you should never compromise your values just for the sake of your image. For example, most people wouldn't buy a car they can't afford because they think it would make them look prosperous. The information about your personal life is mentioned here just to give you an idea of how those decisions affect the total picture others may have of you. Of course, those impressions vary from person to person according to their personalities and past experiences with you and others.

You can influence your image only by what you do now. You couldn't choose your parents; nor can you alter anything you've done or not done in the past. That is why the image you present is so important. It's the only action you can take to shape the impression others have of you.

Contrary to popular notions, first impressions do occur over and over. You are able to correct your image, much as a sailor adjusts the sail when the wind changes. This is not to suggest that you are blown about by every nuance of change, but rather that you have the opportunity to improve your image—and thus your influence.

Image is cumulative as well. Poor impressions linger, in particular. That's the reason first impressions are emphasized. Think about a meeting or class that you attended recently at which you knew several of the participants. Didn't you already know something about what they would say and how they would behave? Accept the paradox that you can't change any previous impressions people have of you but you can add positive impressions now and in the future.

PERCEPTION OF NURSES

"Perception is truth" is a marketing axiom. It is as applicable for nursing as it is for cars, soup, or pharmaceuticals. The general perception of nurses is one-dimensional and inaccurate. Most nurses have heard comments such as, "I could never do what you do; I can't stand blood" and "But I'm glad you're doing it." Although nurses constitute the majority of health care professionals, they are largely invisible. Their competence, skill, knowledge, and judgment are—as the word "image" suggests—only a reflection, not reality.

Public Perception of Nurses

Although the public ranks nurses highest on honesty and ethics (Gallup, 2010), nursing ranks low in career desirability, numbering 100 out of 250 and below respiratory therapists, physician's assistants, and podiatrists (Strieber, 2010). In addition, the ranking, conducted by Career Cast (http://www.careercast.com), states that a registered nurse, "*Assists* physicians in administering holistic medical care and treatment to assigned patients in clinics, hospitals, public health centers, and health maintenance organizations" (emphasis added). Even a company that publishes job advertisements misstates nurses' work.

How members of the public perceive nurses is related to their experiences with nurses. If they've been a patient or observed a family member receiving nursing care and if they were impressed by that care, they tend to retain a positive impression of all nurses. Similarly, people have a positive image of nursing if they have a friend or relative who is a nurse and who has talked about the rewards and satisfaction of being a nurse. If, on the other hand, experiences with nurses have been negative or they have heard nurses say they regret being a nurse, their opinions will be less favorable. Generally, though, nurses remain the invisible majority in health care, and the public has few impressions of nurses, positive or negative.

Media Image of Nursing

The media has been accused of perpetuating nursing's poor public image, but in reality, the media simply reflect public opinion of nurses' work, no matter how much nurses are trusted. Nurses have often failed to take advantage of the opportunity to respond to media requests for information, saying such things as, "You'll have to ask the doctor" even when the query relates to nursing care. (See Chapter 12 for information on ways to interact with the media.)

Institutions also perpetuate this erroneous image. In her blog, Suzanne Gordon rails against an ad for New York University's Langone Medical Center that had recently been awarded Magnet Status (Gordon, 2010). Expecting the ad to promote this newly bestowed recognition, Gordon was sadly disappointed. Only doctors were featured in the ad, the implication being that it is only the presence of doctors that ensures safe care—despite the IOM report more than a decade ago about the appalling rate of medical mistakes (Institute of Medicine, 1999).

The TV shows *Grey's Anatomy*, *House*, and *Private Practice* topped The Truth in Nursing's 2010 worst media portrayals of nurses (Nurse.com, 2011). In these shows, nurses are depicted as silent or surly handmaidens to doctors, who frequently yell at them. On *Grey's Anatomy*, for example, doctors perform nursing functions (passing medications, identifying a failing patient, calling a code, and so on) while nurses sit at a nurses station or simply hand the doctors instruments, reports, or equipment.

Other media portrayals that reflect poorly on nursing include Mariah Carey dressed as a nurse in a music video, Helen Mirren's comment on the *Late Show with David Letterman* suggesting that prostitutes come from nursing because "they're used to naked bodies," and a segment on the *Dr. Oz Show* in which Mehmet Oz danced with women attired in sexy nurse outfits to promote dancing as a weight-loss strategy (The Truth About Nursing Awards, 2011).

On the other hand, The Truth in Nursing cited *Nurse Jackie* as one of the best media portrayals of nurses (2011). The character, Jackie Peyton, is a flawed but competent, knowledgeable, and skilled nurse. She fights for her patients, stands up to the administrator and physicians, battles the bureaucracy, and shows compassion to both patients and families.

Two mystery book authors, Anne Perry and Charles Todd, portray strong nurse characters in their fiction. Anne Perry's William Monk series features Hester Latterly, an 1860s independent nurse in England, and Charles

Todd's Bess Crawford series features a courageous World War I nurse. The protagonist in my own mysteries is a confident, compassionate nurse, created to show nurses' work and the setting accurately. (See the Web Resources section later in this chapter for links to these authors' books.)

Why Nursing's Image Matters

A negative image of nursing affects us all (Summers & Summers, 2010). Lack of support from administrators, physicians, and the public shapes nurses' beliefs in themselves and their colleagues. They may burn out, act out, or leave the profession. Furthermore, such stereotypes discourage potential recruits.

What nurses do contributes directly to patients' goals and outcomes. Every nurse knows that, but few acknowledge it publicly. Describing the actions you took to care for a patient is not bragging (as some nurses think); it is simply an account of your work.

Nursing is a service profession but not a subservient one. Pilots are an example of service without servility; nurses can do the same. Pride in your work, yourself, and your profession can translate into actions that help you present yourself positively. All of us want to know that when we need a nurse, he or she will be there. And each one of us contributes to that image by the way that we present ourselves.

PRESENTING A POSITIVE IMAGE

By now, you should understand how important your image is in helping you become more influential and contributing to a positive image of nursing. The way in which you introduce yourself, how you perform your work, and how you acknowledge the patient outcomes that are attributable to nurses' actions all affect the image the public has of nurses.

How can you present the best image of yourself and your profession? A clean, well-groomed appearance is a given to project a positive image of yourself and nursing (Pagana, 2010). Anything that draws attention away from your professionalism should be avoided. Examples include jangling jewelry, visible tattoos, multiple piercings, and long fingernails. Evaluating your behavior, including your posture, use of gestures, language (e.g., choice of words, manner of speaking, errors in grammar), and your command of proper etiquette is essential before you can decide what you wish to improve. (See Chapter 11 for advanced skills in presenting yourself.)

We all have room for improvement, but objectively examining ourselves is difficult. More important, it takes a concerted effort to change lifelong habits. Only people who truly want to enhance their image will be able to do so, and then it will remain an ongoing project.

Image in Specific Settings

How you present yourself varies according to the setting, the circumstances, your audience, and your goal. In work settings, you want to present an image of professionalism, using your positional, expert, and informational power. You interact with patients and their families, coworkers, students, assistive personnel, physicians, administrators, instructors, and many others in the course of your work. Everyone in your sphere of work will have an impression of you. How they see you will influence their opinion not only of you but of nursing as a whole.

At a nursing association meeting, your image might be more collegial. You're with people who have much in common with you, so your goal might be to gather information or to become more involved in the organization.

In community settings, such as a parent-teacher organization at your child's school or a neighborhood association meeting, you will have other goals. You might want to learn about a new math curriculum or changes in zoning laws. There, too, you are presenting your image. Your outward appearance reflects your inner qualities, and your image as a competent professional should predominate.

Image Detractors

Examples of image detractors are shown in Table 4-2. Fortunately, these are amenable to change. Don't dress to distract. Help people focus on you, not your accessories. Evaluate yourself honestly and make every effort to change those aspects of your appearance that detract from your professional image.

Etiquette and grammar also affect image. Using both correctly conveys an image of confidence and competence. If you are unsure how well your manners and language portray that image, review business etiquette or grammar sites online. Also, watch others to see how they conduct themselves, such as the way they introduce people, and—even more important—watch their table manners. Model their example. Additionally, you can ask a close friend or family member to report if they notice lapses in your manners or grammar. The most common problems people have with grammar is saying, for example, "Him and I went to the store" instead of "He and I went to the store."

TABLE 4-2 Image Detractors
Excessive weight
Poor posture
Extreme mannerisms
Obscene or inappropriate language
Incorrect grammar
Visible tattoos, piercings
Poor personal hygiene
Clothing unclean, unpressed, or in disrepair
Fingernails excessively long or decorated
Smoking, drinking, drugs
Nail biting and other offensive personal habits

What You Know Now

You have learned that your image consists of the sum total of how you present yourself. You know that the perception most people have of nurses and the work they do is inaccurate, unseen, and unknown. You learned that you can change your own image to reflect the professional nurse that you are. You know that you can contribute to the public's image of nursing by how you dress and how you conduct yourself in various situations.

Begin now to let your image reflect the confident and competent professional that you are!

Tools for Image

1. Identify ways in which nurses present a positive image.
2. Apply your nursing skills of observation to your own image.
3. Incorporate the positive attributes of nurses into your own self-image. Remind yourself of these daily.
4. Remember that the way you present yourself conveys an image of you and your profession that goes with you everywhere.

Learning Activities

1. Close your eyes and imagine yourself in the image you desire. Open your eyes and make a plan to make that image real. Share your plan with a friend or a class.
2. Study an etiquette book or website, paying special attention to business ethics. Practice those skills at every opportunity. Report to your class or share your experiences with a friend.
3. During a one-week period, try to find all the news articles about health care in print, radio, and television. Identify subjects about which nurses could supply information, such as adopting a diabetic regimen. Think about ways you could communicate that information to the media. Keep your ideas to use after you read Chapter 11.

References

Gallup. (2010). In U.S., more than 8 in 10 rate nurses, doctors highly. Retrieved January 20, 2011, from http://www.gallup.com/poll/145214/Rate-Nurses-Doctors-Highly.aspx

Gordon, S. (March 13, 2010). *NYU Langone Medical Center and Nursing Image.* Retrieved October 15, 2010, from http://www.suzannegordon.com/?m=201003

Institute of Medicine (1999). *To err is human: Building a safer health system.* Retrieved October 15, 2010, from http://www.nap.edu/openbook.php?record_id=9728

LaSala, K. B., & Nelson, J. (2005). What contributes to professionalism. *MEDSURG Nursing, 14*(1), 63–67.

Nurse.com. (2011). Nonprofit group highlights best, worst nurse portrayals in pop culture. Retrieved April 18, 2011, from http://news.nurse.com/article/20110106/NATIONAL02/101170004/-1/frontpage

Pagana, K. D. (2010). 7 tips to improve your professional etiquette. *Nursing Management, 41*(5), 45–48.

Strieber, A. (2010). *The top 200 jobs of 2010.* Retrieved online at http://www.careercast.com/jobs/content/top-200-job-ranking-5

Summers, S., & Summers, H. J. (2009). *Saving lives: Why the media portrayal of nurses puts us all at risk.* New York: Kaplan Publishing.

Thomas, C. M., Ehret, A., Ellis, B., Colon-Shoop, S., Linton, J., & Metz, S. (2010). Perception of nurse caring, skills, and knowledge based on appearance. *Journal of Nursing Administration, 40*(11), 489–497.

Truth About Nursing Awards. (2011). The 2010 truth about nursing awards. Retrieved January 18, 2011, from http://www.truthaboutnursing.org/press/awards/2010/awd

Web Resources

Hitti, M. Nurses' images in movies improving. Retrieved April 15, 2011, from http://www.medscape.com/viewarticle/581973

Sullivan, E. J. Why nursing? *Journal of Professional Nursing, 16*(3). Retrieved April 15, 2011, from http://www.eleanorsullivan.com/pdf/whynursing.pdf

Yox, S. Nurses should play greater role in health policy. Retrieved April 15, 2011, from http://boards.medscape.com/forums?128@239.OKdtai1BGTy@.29fa124e!comment=1

For nursing mysteries, see: http://www.anneperry.net, http://www.charlestodd.com, and http://www.EleanorSullivan.com

Print Resource

Post, P., & Post, P. (2005). *Emily Post's the etiquette advantage in business: Personal skills for professional success* (2nd ed.). New York: William Morrow.

CASE STUDY

Improving Image

Anna and Selena both enjoyed participating in their local chapter of the Emergency Room Nurses Association, attending monthly meetings, and serving on subcommittees and work groups.

At one monthly meeting, Anna noticed that Selena dressed as she usually did, in dress slacks, a button-down shirt, and her hospital ID badge. Because they both regularly requested the day off to attend, Anna thought it was silly to "dress up" for the Friday meeting. Instead, Anna wore her St. Mercy Hospital sweatshirt and jeans to the meetings so that everyone would know where she worked and so that she could run errands after the meetings.

The discussion turned to teaching community classes about using bike helmets and seat belt use. "Your thoughts?" the president asked Selena. Anna had an idea about that subject too, but the president ignored her raised hand. In fact, she realized, people often sought Selena's opinions and ideas. Why was she approached so often when Anna was rarely asked for suggestions? Anna had actually worked in the emergency room for three years longer than Selena!

Anna looked around the room. It dawned on her that the people who were making the most contributions were all dressed in professional business attire. Whatever the topic, these nurses' ideas were incorporated into the discussion.

Anna vowed to change her appearance for the meetings. They were, after all, professional occasions that required appropriate attire.

At the next meeting, Anna wore a gray skirt and wool sweater with her hospital ID badge. As soon as she entered the room, Anna saw that people approached her expectantly. Then several active members seated themselves near her.

When the discussion turned to ways to improve patients' waiting room experiences, the president turned to Anna. "How is your ER managing patients who need to be admitted when no beds are available?"

Anna smiled. This was what she'd been waiting for.

5

Communicating Effectively

Don't interrupt me when I'm interrupting you.

WINSTON CHURCHILL

In this chapter, you will learn:

- How communication affects influence
- How your behavior speaks louder than your words
- How men and women communicate differently
- How to improve your communication skills

COMMUNICATION DEFINED

Communication is the process of interacting with two or more individuals or groups. Communication can be verbal or nonverbal, but most communication is a combination of both verbal and nonverbal messages. Verbal communication includes all aspects of language: words, grammar, style, and content. Nonverbal communication, however, is more powerful than spoken words. It communicates the message behind the message, that is, what the person really means.

It's not what we say; it's how we say it.

Tone of voice, facial expression, dress, body language, gestures, eye contact, handshakes, silence, and where participants are seated are examples of nonverbal communication. These characteristics frame the verbal message and may communicate a message congruent with the verbal communication or may send a very different message.

"Why is she smiling when she's really mad?" asked a five-year-old child, referring to the store's cashier. The child correctly read the cashier's nonverbal language and understood the message behind the message—the accurate one.

For the Novice Nurse

You don't need this chapter. Or so you think. You've finished school, passed state boards, and have your first job in nursing. And you've been communicating all your life. But don't be too quick to dismiss the content presented here. Read it, think about it, and then decide if communication isn't more complicated than you thought.

It is!

EFFECTIVE COMMUNICATION

Nurses use communication with patients and their families, coworkers, superiors, subordinates, and other health care providers. Nurses communicate with colleagues in their profession and represent nursing in their communities. Being able to communicate effectively is essential for nurses to become influential.

Communication, however, is fraught with opportunities to be misinterpreted and misunderstood for both message sender and receiver over the course of an interaction. Although easier to understand than nonverbal signals, even written communication can be misinterpreted. Box 5-1 shows how the meaning of words, although accurate, can be distorted.

Nonverbal communication is frequently misunderstood, generally because people attend to the words and not the message behind the message—even if the sender and receiver do not see each other. Tone of voice, inflection, and the length of the message are examples of nonverbal communication conveyed by voice mail, for example. E-mail messages are also often misconstrued. Even when participants are communicating in person, nonverbal messages—especially if they are incongruent with the verbal message—often are discounted or ignored.

Additionally, the context, the setting, the purpose, the past experiences, and the presence of observers all affect communication. Discussing communication in depth is beyond the scope of this book; simply stated, communication is effective when the message the sender intends and the receiver understands are congruent. This statement holds true whether the message is a positive one (e.g., "You did a good job leading that meeting"), negative (e.g., "You're late with this quarter's report"), or neutral (e.g., "Think it will rain today?"). Many factors can interfere with accurate understanding of messages sent and received, including cultural influences, the relative status of each (e.g., supervisor and staff nurse), and gender differences. (See Chapter 11 for information on understanding the meaning behind the message.)

BOX 5-1

Distorted Communication

There is ample opportunity for distortion in the complicated process of sending, receiving, and responding to messages, as demonstrated by the following correspondence between a plumber and an official of the National Bureau of Standards.

Bureau of Standards
Washington, D.C.
Gentlemen:
I have been in the plumbing business for over 11 years and have found that hydrochloric acid works real fine for cleaning drains. Could you tell me if it's harmless?
Sincerely
Tom Brown, Plumber

Mr. Tom Brown, Plumber
Yourtown, U.S.A.
Dear Mr. Brown:
We wish to inform you we have your letter of last week and advise that we cannot assume responsibility for the production of toxic and noxious residues with hydrochloric acid and further suggest you use an alternate procedure.
Sincerely,
Bureau of Standards

Mr. Tom Brown, Plumber
Yourtown, U.S.A.
Dear Mr. Brown:
The efficacy of hydrochloric acid is indisputable, but the chlorine residue is incompatible with metallic permanence!
Sincerely,
Bureau of Standards

Bureau of Standards
Washington, D.C.
Gentlemen:
I have your most recent letter and am happy to find you still agree with me.
Sincerely,
Tom Brown, Plumber

Bureau of Standards
Washington, D.C.
Gentlemen:
I have your letter of last week and am mightily glad you agree with me on the use of hydrochloric acid.
Sincerely,
Tom Brown, Plumber

Mr. Tom Brown, Plumber
Yourtown, U.S.A.
Dear Mr. Brown:
Don't use hydrochloric acid, it eats the hell out of pipes!
Sincerely,
Bureau of Standards

For communication among more than two people, the chance of distortion increases proportionally.

Sullivan, E. J. (2013). *Effective leadership and management in nursing* (8th ed.). Upper Saddle River, NJ: Prentice Hall Health.

Social Media Communication

Social media has revolutionized communication in just the last few years (Kaplan & Haenlein, 2010). Social media encourages collaboration and the exchange of images, ideas, opinions, and preferences in networking websites, online forums, weblogs, social blogs, wikis, podcasts, RSS feeds, photos, video content communities, social bookmarking, online chat rooms, microblogs such as Twitter, and social media communities such as Facebook and LinkedIn.

Similar to other enterprises, most health care organizations have an online presence with a website and social media sites such as Facebook, Twitter, and blogs. Units within the organization may have Facebook pages as well, with staff able to post on those sites. These opportunities for information sharing and relationship building come with risk as well (Raso, 2010; Trossman, 2010). Patient confidentiality, the organization's reputation, and recruiting efforts can be enhanced or put in jeopardy by posts to the site. (See the case study at the end of this chapter.)

Gender Differences in Communication

The workplace is fraught with opportunities for miscommunication, including those between men and women (Helgesen & Johnson, 2010). Linguist Deborah Tannen explored these differences in the communication styles of men and women in her very popular book *Talking from 9 to 5* (1994). Women, she suggests, tend to work toward consensus, soften negative comments, and avoid boasting about their own accomplishments. As a result, men often see women as unable to make decisions, manipulative, or weak.

Men use communication rituals such as banter and playful put-downs to avoid appearing in a lower position. Women may take these conversational strategies literally. When women attempt to take everyone's feelings into consideration, men see them as less competent than they are. Like the rules discussed in Chapter 2, both men and women must recognize differences in each other's styles of communication and strive toward gender-neutral interactions. (See Tables 5-1 and 5-2).

Neither men nor women should raise their voices—no matter what the provocation. Nor should you omit important details or assume that everyone knows what you mean. Not allowing questions or objections also should be avoided. Never walk away and talk at the same time (Donaldson, 2007).

TABLE 5-1 Gender Differences in Communication

Men tend to	Women tend to
Interrupt more frequently	Wait to be noticed
Talk more, longer, louder, and faster	Use qualifiers (prefacing and tagging)
Disagree more	Use questions in place of statements
Focus on the issue more than the person	Relate personal experiences
Boast about accomplishments	Promote consensus
Use banter to avoid an inferior position	Withdraw from conflict

TABLE 5-2 Recommendations for Gender-Neutral Communication

Men may need to	Women may need to
Listen to objections and suggestions	State their message clearly and concisely
Listen without feeling responsible	Solve problems without personalizing them
Suspend judgment until information is in	Say what they want without hinting
Explain their reasons	Eliminate unsure words ("sort of") and nonwords ("truly")
Don't yell	Don't cry

Active Listening

Active listening requires more than silence while others are talking (Boynton, 2009; Post & Post, 2005). The following steps help turn passive listening into active listening:

1. Stay in the present, mentally and emotionally.
2. Don't interrupt. Let the other party finish sentences, but do make occasional acknowledgements with a nod or "okay."
3. Ask questions to clarify or reflect on the speaker's statements.
4. Pay attention to every word, gesture, tone of voice, and silence. Take notes if appropriate, especially if listening on the phone.
5. Think about what the speaker said, what it means in the context of the conversation and the issue, and how it reflects on your future relationship.

Barriers to Effective Listening

Most nurses believe they are good listeners. Observing and listening to patients are skills nurses learn early in their careers and use every day. Being a good listener, however, involves more than just hearing words and watching body language. Maintaining eye contact is misleading; it may or may not

BOX 5-2
Listening to Body Language

Listening	Not Listening
Smiling	Blank look
Eye contact	Teeth clenched
Arms spread	Arms crossed over chest
Hands open or touching face	Hand over mouth
Leaning forward	Leaning back or head tilted away

signal that a person is listening. (See Box 5-2.) Barriers to effective listening include preconceived beliefs, lack of self-confidence, flagging energy, defensiveness, and habit (Donaldson, 2007).

PRECONCEIVED BELIEFS. The older your relationship with someone is, the more apt you are to think you know what the person says or means, and thus the more likely you are to not listen. This rule holds true in personal as well as professional relationships and applies to groups of people (known as stereotyping, as mentioned earlier). Not expecting others to have anything worthwhile to say is also an example of preconceptions about them. Some men, especially in work settings, tend to view women in this way.

LACK OF SELF-CONFIDENCE. Listening is difficult if you are nervous, and weak self-confidence is frequently the cause. People tend to talk too much or think about what they're planning to say next too much to pay attention to the person speaking. Often their mind is racing, and they may not be listening even when they're talking themselves.

FLAGGING ENERGY. Listening takes energy; sometimes we simply don't have enough to listen carefully. Too many people speaking at once, too much to do, being worried, or being too tired can all interfere with our ability to listen.

DEFENSIVENESS. Survival required that we learn to hear danger approaching, but today humans have translated defense mechanisms into a way to avoid hearing bad news. Then, we think, we don't have to deal with it. The opposite, however, is true. Only when we can hear and consider information can we handle it.

HABIT. Over time, many people develop the habit of thinking ahead during conversations. Thinking ahead is valuable in most aspects of life, but it's deadly when you need to be listening. People speaking to you can tell you're not listening (can't you?), but they will seldom tell you so, especially if you have higher status than they do. Like all behaviors that have become habits, changing this one is not easy. Reminding yourself to refocus on the speaker can help.

ENHANCING YOUR COMMUNICATION SKILLS

All communication occurs within the context of a relationship, the environment, and your purpose. What you say and how you say it varies if you are requesting help, speaking to your boss, or listening to directions. Communication differs if it is one-on-one, takes place informally, occurs in a structured meeting and based on whether you initiate the communication, are a member of a group, or lead an organizational meeting. Numerous other configurations of communication occur as well. Selecting the appropriate medium to use is one of the first steps in improving your communication skills.

Choosing the Medium

We can communicate with others in person, by phone, by text, by e-mail, by fax, by postal mail, and by leaving voice mail messages. Selecting the appropriate medium based on the person and your purpose is essential to communicate effectively. Each medium serves a specific purpose. In general, the more important the information, the closer you should be to the recipient.

IN PERSON. One-on-one contact is required for messages that need clarification, are sensitive, or are confidential. Terminating employment is an example. Individuals can see and hear each other with much less likelihood of distortion when they are together. Questions can be asked and answered and understanding is more likely to occur.

PHONE. Phone conversations are one step removed from in-person communications. There, too, tone of voice, inflection, and nuances of speech can be heard and questions can be asked. Particularly if you know the person well or the subject is not controversial, telephone contact is less time-consuming than a personal meeting and may be the best choice in this situation. However, remember that cell phone conversations may be overheard and confidentiality cannot be guaranteed (Pagana, 2009).

VOICE MAIL. Voice mail allows people to leave messages and receive responses at their convenience, which is especially helpful for busy people and for those in different time zones. A message is one more step removed from meeting with someone in person. It is appropriate for providing requested information or communicating when and where a meeting is scheduled, for example.

Messages should be kept short and to the point. Your voice should be warm, inviting, and business-like. It helps to plan what you are going to say before calling, regardless of whether you're speaking to the person or leaving a message. Jotting down a few notes helps if the issue is important or sensitive. Decide beforehand whether you need a call back to discuss the topic or if a message will suffice. Be sure to think about how the recipient will hear the message, not just what you want to say. Also realize that someone other than your intended recipient may hear the message.

E-MAIL. E-mail messages have all the attributes of voice mail; in addition, many people can be contacted simultaneously. Routine information or requests for scheduling are examples of the appropriate use of e-mail. Keep in mind that your message may be forwarded to others—do not include highly personal or confidential information, which should be communicated in person, by phone, or (if appropriate) in a letter.

TEXT MESSAGES. Because they are always short, text messages can be easily misinterpreted. Consider your words and their tone before you hit send.

SOCIAL MEDIA. Social media sites, such as Facebook, LinkedIn, Twitter, and blogs are invaluable communication tools today for both individuals and organizations. Think about your target audience and how your posts might be seen by others. Remember, too, that whatever you write could exist online forever. Avoid sending text or images that might hinder a future job prospect, hamper a promotion, or damage your relationship with colleagues.

WRITTEN CORRESPONDENCE. Written communication is the farthest medium of delivery from personal communication. Notes are informal; letters are more official. Both serve a purpose, and often written communication is used to follow up after verbal exchanges. Formal letters may be necessary for legal documentation as well.

Because so much communication is now automated, handwritten notes lend a personal touch to the message. Sending a thank-you note is impressive in today's busy world, leaves a positive reflection of you, and can help foster your relationship (Post & Post, 2005).

All of these forms of communication offer a multitude of opportunities for distortion and miscommunication. Only by carefully considering your message, the recipient, and the purpose can you decide which forms to use.

Crafting Your Message

The content of your message varies according to your relationship to the receiver (e.g., your boss versus your auto mechanic), the setting (e.g., your office or theirs), and the purpose (e.g., ask for a raise, give instructions for a task).

STRIVE FOR CLARITY. Determining your goal in the communication is the first step toward clarity. This helps to keep the other person from admonishing you to "get to the point." By then it's too late to be clear. Following are the steps to craft a clear message:

1. ***State your goal in one sentence.*** Write it down if necessary. Will it make sense to the person to whom you plan to send it? Rework it until you have your goal clearly in your mind.
2. ***Craft an overview paragraph.*** You can do this in your mind if it's short. If you need to remember more, jot down your main points in descending order of importance. Be accurate. If you don't know something, try to find out ahead of time or be prepared to admit that you don't know if asked.
3. ***Consider what the other person might say in response to each point.*** Try to think of how to answer and possibly incorporate objections into your message. Don't overdo this step, though; you might be inadvertently arguing against your own ideas.
4. ***Be prepared to listen carefully to the response.*** Are objections valid? Can you overcome them or modify your goal? If you are interrupted or

your recipient is distracted, you may decide to delay the interaction. Remember what has been said and, if it's important, make a few notes to trigger your thoughts later.

BARRIERS TO CLARITY. Some of the reasons that people fail to make themselves clear are a fear of rejection, a lack of concentration, or an unwillingness to confront a problem (Donaldson, 2007). A rejection of your ideas is not a rejection of you, but the two are often confused. By being vague and leaving conclusions unsaid, people think they can avoid rejection, but the opposite is true. By the time the other person finally understands what you were saying, you may have lost your hoped-for support.

Losing concentration is another impediment to clarity (Griffin, 2008). When you know the message and know where you want the discussion to go, it's easy to let your mind wander. Don't let it. Focusing on your recipient and listening carefully can help counter the tendency to lose concentration.

We all like to be liked, and confronting someone with a problem carries the chance of damaging someone's good opinion of us. Being clear in such a situation is even more important. If we're unclear, we're only postponing the inevitable bad news and weakening our status overall. We are doing the person no favors by avoiding negative information; it's often worse later. Deliver bad news with respect for the dignity of the person, and maintain your composure regardless of the person's response.

Related to confronting a person with a problem is the unenviable task of saying no to a request, which also carries hazards to relationships. Three steps can make saying no more palatable (Donaldson, 2007). First, acknowledge the person and the request, as in, "I can see this equipment request is important to help you do your job." Next, describe your situation, as in, "Unfortunately, I just had a budget cut and I have to decide on priorities for the unit." Finally, convey your decision, as in, "I can't authorize this now, but I'd be glad to put it at the top of the list for next year." You've acknowledged the person and the importance of the request, you've shown that you've considered the request, and you've made the best decision you could under the circumstances.

Delivering Your Message

Poor delivery can undermine the best-worded message. Using qualifiers, such as "I'm sure you've thought of this" or "I don't know if you'd be interested" to preface your message diminishes its importance before anyone has heard your ideas. Adding tags after your message, such as "Am I right?" does the same.

Using questions instead of statements makes you sound uncertain, and your listeners are apt to feel the same. Qualifiers such as "sort of" or "kind of" also reduce the effectiveness of your message, and nonwords like "really" and "truly" detract as well. State your message clearly, directly, and with confidence. You are a respected colleague on the health care team. Let your delivery style reflect that belief.

Timing

Timing plays an important role in deciding what to say and how to say it. A discharge conference with a patient's family is a scheduled event, and participants know why they are there, so choosing your words is easier than, for example, trying to catch your boss as she's leaving to ask for time off. In the latter case, a better option might be to ask for a meeting later. Many opportunities for successful communications have been lost because of poor timing.

Asking Questions

Listening attentively and asking the right questions help you gain knowledge and understanding. It is the best way to counter vague and ambiguous messages. Eliciting facts and obtaining opinions are the two reasons to ask questions. Just as there are skills to crafting message, so are there skills to constructing questions. Think of questions as building blocks on the topic, and use them to construct a structure of the issue. Here are some suggestions to make your questions garner the information you want (Donaldson, 2007):

1. Decide what information you want. Is it facts or opinion?
2. Adapt the question to the speaker, using words and examples appropriate to the person.
3. Ask general questions first; follow up with more specific ones.
4. Stick to one subject at a time.
5. Avoid leading questions.
6. Don't assume that you know the speaker's intent; ask for clarification.
7. Ask open-ended questions.

Sometimes people use questions to intimidate others. When that happens, no answer is the best response. Silence is a powerful tool, but it takes strength and patience. "The next person who talks loses" is an old sales adage. Remember it.

Using Interruptions

Interrupting is a communication strategy that can be used to support or to counteract and undermine. Interruptions can be affirming: "I agree" and "absolutely" are examples. Or, they can be used to attack the speaker or the message. Holding the floor and not allowing anyone else to talk is rude and can lead the more assertive (or frustrated) people to interrupt. Some people even interrupt themselves, jumping from one thought to another. Be alert to how you and others use interruptions and be sure to use them appropriately.

What You Know Now

You have learned that effective communication includes how your message affects your intended receivers—and possibly others. You learned that listening involves people's words and nonverbal behaviors as well as your relationship and the situation. You understand that men and women tend to communicate differently and that both must strive toward gender-neutral communications. You realize the impact that social media has on communication and how to use such sites appropriately. You learned some communication strategies, including how to select the appropriate medium, how to craft your message, and how to deliver it effectively.

All set? Let's talk!

Tools for Effective Communication

1. Observe influential people to see how they communicate.
2. Think about what you are going to say; try to be as accurate and concise as you can.
3. Pay attention to body language—yours and others.
4. Cultivate active listening habits.
5. Learn to use social media appropriately.
6. Chose the best medium, craft clear messages, and deliver them appropriately.

Learning Activities

1. Recall your experience described in the activity in Chapter 1. Role-play the same situation using the skills included in this chapter.
2. Observe participants in a meeting. See if you can discover the message they are going to deliver before they speak. Observe, for example, how people enter the room, where and how they are seated, their body language, and what you know about them from previous experiences, if any. See how accurate you are. Now examine where and how you are seated, your body language, and what the others know about you. Do your words match your nonverbal signals?
3. Use your voice mail for this activity.
   a. Make three calls to your own phone and record your messages as follows: (1) offer some information; (2) ask a favor; and (3) report some bad news (nothing serious). Listen to your messages. What message did you convey? Was it what you intended? Did your voice fit the message?
   b. Call again and listen to your outgoing message. Does it communicate the image you would like? Change it if it doesn't. One hint: smile while you're recording. Share your messages with a colleague or class and ask for their feedback. See if their opinions differ from yours.
4. How clear are you? Think of a recent personal or professional communication that you initiated. Then ask yourself:
   a. What did you want to accomplish with this interaction?
   b. Did you say what you planned to say?
   c. Did you state your goals clearly?
   d. Did you listen and respond to questions and comments?
   e. Did you use an appropriate medium (e.g., over the phone, via e-mail, in person)?
   f. Did you achieve the outcome that you intended?
   g. What would you do differently next time?

References

Boynton, B. (2009). How to improve your listening skills. *American Nurse Today, 4*(9), 50–51.

Donaldson, M. C. (2007). *Negotiating for dummies* (2nd ed.). New York: Wiley Publishing.

Griffin, J. (2008). *How to say it at work: Putting yourself across with power words, phrases, body language and communication secrets* (2nd ed.). Paramus, NJ: Prentice Hall Press.

Helgesen, S., & Johnson, J. (2010). *The female vision: Women's real power at work.* San Francisco: Berrett-Koehler Publications.

Kaplan, A. M., & Haenlein, M. (2010). Users of the world, unite! The challenges and opportunities of social media. *Business Horizons, 53*(1), 59–68.

Pagana, K. D. (2009). A user's guide to cell-phone etiquette. *American Nurse Today, 4*(3), 36–37.

Post, P., & Post, P. (2005). *Emily Post's the etiquette advantage in business: Personal skills for professional success* (2nd ed.). New York: William Morrow.

Raso, R. (2010). Social media for nurse managers: What does it all mean? *Nursing Management, 41*(8), 23–25.

Tannen, D. (1994). *Talking from 9 to 5: How women's and men's conversational styles affect who gets heard, who gets credit, and what gets done at work.* New York: Morrow.

Trossman, S. (2010). Sharing too much? Nurses nationwide need more information on social networking pitfalls. *American Nurse Today, 5*(11), 38–39.

Web Resources

Anderson, L. L. Communication in nursing. Retrieved April 15, 2011, from http://www.nursetogether.com/tabid/102/itemid/906/Communication-in-Nursing.aspx

Lindsay, C. Two-way street: Open line of communication between nurses and managers helps maintain staff strength. Retrieved April 15, 2011, from http://www.nurseweek.com/news/features/01-03/twoway.asp

Arford, P. H. Nurse-physician communication: An organizational accountability. Retrieved April 15, 2011, from http://www.medscape.com/viewarticle/502806

Print Resource

Post, P., & Post, P. (2005). *Emily Post's the etiquette advantage in business: Personal skills for professional success* (2nd ed.). New York: William Morrow.

CASE STUDY

Sharing Information

Zachary led the social committee on his oncology patient care unit. The committee planned potlucks, quarterly birthday parties, holiday gatherings, and community service activities. In order to communicate in as many ways as possible, activities were e-mailed, posted on bulletin boards, sent via text message, and posted online on the unit's social networking page.

One day, a longtime leukemia patient, Mrs. Bright, died after becoming septic. Though she had been only 39 years old, Mrs. Bright had been a regular patient on the oncology unit for more than five years, and the staff had grown close to her and her three young sons and husband.

Some staff members weren't working that day, and Zachary was certain they'd want to know the sad news. After work that night, he posted the announcement on the unit's social networking site.

The next day at work, Zachary's manager asked to speak with him. "Did you post Mrs. Bright's death on our unit's social networking page?"

"Yes," Zachary answered. "I wanted to be sure that everyone knew about her death because she was such a special patient to the unit."

"I realize your intentions were not malicious and Mrs. Bright's family had told the staff that they could tell everyone about her passing. However, it is inappropriate use of the social networking website page to put any patient information on there. It's not a confidential medium, and it was a violation of the patient's privacy as well."

Zachary apologized for his oversight. "It was a lesson for me to learn."

At next month's staff meeting, Zachary and his manager presented an in-service lecture on the ways in which it was and was not acceptable to use technological information-sharing resources. They wanted to ensure that the same error did not happen again.

6

Why Politics?

Adventures don't begin until you get into the forest.

MICKEY HART,
GRATEFUL DEAD DRUMMER

In this chapter, you will learn:

- What politics means
- How politics is a game (like the rules are)
- How policies evolve from political activities
- Why you need to know political strategies
- How you can become politically savvy

WHAT IS POLITICS, REALLY?

Politics and influence are closely entwined and sometimes confused with each other. Politicians have influence, so influential people are assumed to be political. The word "politics" is often used in a negative context. "Playing politics" refers to nefarious and underhanded means to achieve one's ends, usually at the expense of more deserving others.

Politics, however, is a neutral word. It means the art of influencing others to achieve desirable goals, usually by acquiring resources (Mason, Leavitt, & Chaffee, 2011). Money is the most common resource, but time, space, personnel, equipment, information, and support are examples of other resources sought.

Decisions about resources occur constantly. Should you buy a Lexus or a Kia? Should you leave work early to take your son to soccer practice? Will the new office go to the hospital's vice president for nursing or the chief financial officer? Who will work on the Fourth of July? Which faculty member will teach the foundations course?

The Relationship between Politics and Policy

Policy is the plan that results from political action (see "The Process of Political Action" later in the chapter). Policies are made in governments at the municipal, state, and federal levels, as you know, but policies are made in many other arenas as well. Policies govern health care institutions, universities, places of business, professional associations, community and religious groups, and your home, among other areas. Policies are decided informally (e.g., what time a teenager should be home) but may be more formal (e.g., hospital policies and procedures manual) or even legally enforceable (e.g., sexual harassment policies).

For the Novice Nurse

"I don't do politics," one new nurse said. "My life's too full now." But here's what he didn't know: politics is how decisions are made, and these decisions affect his work and his patients. Starting out, he had an opportunity to observe how policies were made and how they affected the people involved, both positively and negatively. He could see how people worked together or didn't and what resulted. He could learn to become political.

So can you.

The Game of Politics

Just as the world of work is described as a game in Chapter 2, so can politics be viewed as a game (Green & Chaney, 2006). Certain rules apply in one organization but may be different in other settings. The rules identify who can participate, how they participate, when they can be involved, and who referees. Whoever gets the resources is the winner.

> A nursing administrator was recently hired away from a small community hospital to be the vice president of patient care in a large, multi-institutional health care system. Her first priority was to prepare the coming year's budget. She knew that the system had been losing money and her boss had asked her to prepare a budget with a 5 percent reduction from the previous year's.
>
> The administrator had spent her first few weeks getting to know the system and the major players, and determining the adequacy of nurse staffing and the quality of nursing care. She learned that nursing was well-regarded among most senior administrators.

The nursing staff were experienced and competent but coverage was inadequate, mostly due to the nursing shortage. She worried that cutting the staffing budget would result in increased turnover and exacerbate the problem. What could she do?

In her old hospital, she would have gone straight to the hospital administrator and explained the problem. She knew he would have done all he could to help, possibly excusing her from the budget reduction or modifying it. In her current organization, no one hospital administrator could make the final decision about budgets and the demands of offsite clinics, residency programs, a trauma center, and accreditation competed with the funds she needed to at least maintain staffing. Going to the person at the top, chair of the organization's board, was her only option, she thought.

And her first mistake.

The board chair let her know in no uncertain terms that budget decisions were made through the organizational channels and that he would not discuss budgets with her. Furthermore, he expected to never see her making an end run around her supervisors again, or. . . .

You get the picture.

This nursing administrator had learned the game rules in that organization, albeit the hard way.

Nurses have multiple opportunities to use political action skills (also called lobbying) to acquire resources to improve patient care, increase the profession's ability to improve health, and enhance their communities. Vying for scarce resources (e.g., time, money, space, equipment) in the workplace requires savvy political skills.

Politics determines the goals of an organization, such as a professional nursing association or collective bargaining unit. Community groups, including religious organizations, schools (your own or your children's), volunteer groups, and charitable associations, for example, are guided by the political abilities of their members. Groups may expand around the globe (e.g., Sigma Theta Tau International, Rotary International) or may be as limited as a neighborhood association. Nevertheless, their activities are decided by the political skills of their members and leaders.

Learning how to influence policy begins with understanding the process of political action.

THE PROCESS OF POLITICAL ACTION

The political action process is similar to the nursing process; each step determines the next one (see Table 6-1).

First, decide what you or your group want. You are the nurse manager of the renal transplant unit in a large, university medical center. Although

TABLE 6-1 Steps in Political Action

1. Determine what you want.
2. Learn about the players and what they want.
3. Gather supporters and form coalitions.
4. Be prepared to answer opponents.
5. Explain how what you want can help them.

you are fully staffed (at least for the moment!), you realize that valuable staff time is being lost when employees use the Internet for personal use.

You've tried asking employees to desist, but they argue that in the age of technology, it's silly to restrict its use. Besides, they work 12-hour shifts and when a few moments become available, they want to take care of a personal matter. "Furthermore," one staff member told you, "no one should babysit my time."

How much are you willing to compromise? Would you be satisfied if Internet use was restricted to break times? You don't have to know all the alternatives at this point, but be aware that recommendations to modify your plan might be made. Be prepared to consider them.

Second, learn about the players and what they want. Administration wants a sufficient number of employees to care for its patients. With a policy restricting Internet use, they might worry about staff turnover and future hiring problems.

On the other hand, administrators don't want visitors seeing employees using the Internet for personal reasons and thinking it is unprofessional, and they want computers to be available for those needing to complete work activities.

You don't need to ask about anyone's concerns initially. In fact, you don't want to ask about their concerns until you are prepared with enough information to support your proposal. Think about administrators' needs, and you can discover a great deal about their concerns.

Third, gather supporters and form coalitions. Solicit the other nurse managers and charge nurses for their support. Suggest that if a policy were put in place restricting Internet use to work-related purposes, the hospital could monitor patient satisfaction and call light response time to see if satisfaction improves. They could also monitor budgetary savings on technology network investment and staff satisfaction with their coworkers.

Also explain that the money saved from network space could be used for other staff recognition activities, such as an annual hospital picnic or staff T-shirts with the hospital's logo. Describe how such a policy could be presented to managers. If they understand the purposes of the change, they can teach and champion this to their staff. (You will learn more about building coalitions in Chapter 8.)

Fourth, prepare to answer opponents. Talk to information technology staff to ask if personal Internet use puts an undue load on the hospital's network. Meet with patient relations staff to discover if patient satisfaction responses complain about staff personal Internet use or slow call light response time.

You may have discovered what opposition you might face when you thought about the people whose support you need. Talk to a few key people who might have other ideas about opposition to your proposal, but be sure you can trust them to keep your confidence until you are ready to present it. You don't want to build a coalition against you before you've begun.

"Floating a trial balloon" is one way to try out your idea. Ask one or two individuals whose support you would need what they think of the idea. Ask them to be specific. "That would never work," is not enough. Why not? Who would oppose it and why? Are those reasons enough to defeat it?

Fifth, explain how what you want can help them. Administration will be pleased when patients are well cared for. Staff nurses will be ready for report each shift change and can leave on time and not have to stay over. Both administrators and staff will benefit from the better teamwork that may result from a policy that enforces using work time for patient care, not personal business. Also, you could add, money will be available for staff enrichment activities.

Be prepared to compromise, postpone, or abandon your proposal. The support for restricting Internet use to work business only is unreasonable, your colleagues say, with nurses working long hours. It is best to let staff use the Internet on their breaks, a policy that fosters goodwill with them. The managers agree, though, to monitor staff Internet use. You plan to follow up in a few months.

Behind-the-Scenes Work

The effectiveness of any political action is what happens away from the formal meetings. This is known as "behind-the-scenes" work. It is similar to what is necessary to put on a play. The audience doesn't see all that goes on behind the stage before and after the play, but without it, the show couldn't be successfully staged. So it is with political action. You learned some of these strategies in the steps of political action, but there are more.

The "meeting before the meeting" and the "meeting after the meeting" are two more important strategies. The meeting before the meeting encompasses everything that you do ahead of time. You might use this strategy whether you have an item on the agenda or learn beforehand about a topic to be discussed. You may need to talk to people before the meeting to try to discover potential problems before you are asked your opinion. Other people might approach you before the meeting to try to gauge your reaction to their proposal. (They are engaging in their own political action.)

The meeting before the meeting might involve one-on-one interaction, or a few people might get together casually or more formally to prepare for the meeting. The people who live in one neighborhood might meet first to discuss a proposal to change the zoning in their community before the city council meeting.

You might join other nurse managers in the cafeteria and ask their opinions about a personal Internet use policy. This is your opportunity to convince others to support your position, secure their agreement to do so, prepare for their opposition, or to help you decide to delay the issue or to abandon it. Never go into an important meeting that might affect your or others' futures without having had a meeting before the meeting.

The meeting after the meeting offers a chance to consider the discussion that occurred, to strategize about further action, or to compliment a colleague on the way she handled a difficult situation, for example. An additional benefit to meetings before and after scheduled meetings is the opportunity for informal conversations that help build relationships with colleagues.

Dirty Tricks

One especially difficult situation occurs when you have gained someone's support before the meeting but the person does not support you when the meeting occurs. Even before the meeting you may hear that this person is telling other people that he can't support your proposal. This tactic is known as a *dirty trick*. What do you do?

The best strategy is to confront the person directly. "You agreed to support my proposal but now I hear you are speaking against it." Almost inevitably, the person will deny not supporting you. "Oh, no, they misunderstood me. I'm supporting your proposal," is often the response. If this occurs during the meeting or if the person does not speak up to support you as promised, you can use the same tactic: "When we met yesterday, you agreed to support this." You are likely to have her support now that you've confronted her with her deviousness.

There are other reasons, however, for people to change their minds. New information might be presented or they may have thought of other problems. Regardless, they should have told you ahead of time and not allowed you to go into the meeting thinking you still had their support.

New information might come to light during the meeting, and you—as well as your supporters—might change your minds or alter your proposal. Don't be so enamored of your original plan that you become inflexible. You will likely lose, and your rigid position will diminish your influence in the future. (Recall the example of nursing faculty and their conference room in Chapter 2.)

HOW NURSES CAN USE POLITICS

Nurses' political activities began with Florence Nightingale, continued with the emergence of nursing schools and women's suffrage, and improved with the establishment of nursing organizations and the feminist movement.

Nurses are taking their rightful place as politically savvy participants in some spheres of policy making.

Establishing the National Center for Nursing Research (later changed to the National Institute of Nursing Research) within NIH is an example of nurses' powerful political action.

A Brief History of the National Institute of Nursing Research

After the Institute of Medicine report recommended a federal nursing research entity as part of the mainstream scientific community in the early 1980s, nursing leaders in the United States began promoting establishment of a nursing institute at the National Institutes of Health. This effort involved lobbying Congress and the other institutes at NIH—a formidable task. A few members of Congress were interested in the potential that nursing science had for improving health, but the administration was not in favor of another institute at NIH, and the other institutes seemed puzzled about why nursing would need its own institute to do research. Couldn't nurse researchers receive funding through existing institutes? Medicine did so without a separate institute.

Step by step, nursing leaders convinced institute directors and Congress that nursing research would improve human response to illness and assist in maintaining and enhancing health. A bill was born. Concern about cost and increasing bureaucracy emerged and was overcome. The bill passed, only to be vetoed by President Reagan. Then a funny thing happened. Nursing made an unprecedented move. The profession came together, united with one goal: to override President Reagan's veto (none had been successfully overridden before).

One by one, across the country, nurses called their senators and congressional representatives urging support for a nursing institute, explaining that nurses were represented only among a few funded researchers at other institutes who did not understand the impact of nursing interventions on health and recovery. A modest investment, they explained, would yield exponentially greater results. Thanks to a few persuasive members of Congress, a compromise was negotiated and the National Center for Nursing Research was established in 1985. A statutory revision made the Center an Institute in 1993.

Similarly, Georgia nurses successfully changed the state's practice act to include prescriptive authority for advanced practice nurses, overcoming fierce opposition from the medical association (Beall, 2007). Working in concert with each other and with consumers and the media, they generated a letter-writing campaign that countered every obstacle the medical association tried, and Georgia became the last state to grant prescribing privileges to nurse practitioners.

TABLE 6-2 How to Work with Public Officials

1. Be respectful.	5. Understand the issue.
2. Build relationships.	6. Be a constructive opponent.
3. Keep in touch.	7. Be realistic.
4. Arrive informed.	8. Be helpful.

Working with Public Officials

Table 6-2 lists guidelines for working with public officials. First, be respectful. Public officials have many constituents and demands on their support. Build relationships with officials. Don't contact them only when you have a request. Keep in touch at other times.

Communicating with Elected Officials

Nurses often want to contact elected officials to support or oppose legislation. You can call, e-mail, tweet, or write to public officials. (Links to state legislators and contact information for federal government officials are listed in the end-of-chapter Web Resources.)

Here's how to contact state or federal elected officials. Call the official's staff and ask to speak to the person who handles the issue that concerns you. Tell the aide that you support or oppose a certain bill and why. Name the bill by number.

E-mail or write directly to the official. Identify the bill in question, state your position on the bill, and explain why you support or oppose it. Keep your comments brief, and address only one issue per correspondence. Handwritten letters get more attention than form letters distributed by organizations.

Use this format to address members of the U.S. Senate:

The Honorable (full name of senator)
__(Rm.#) __(name of) Senate Office Building
United States Senate
Washington, DC 20510
Dear Senator:

To contact the member of the U.S. Congress, use a similar format:

The Honorable (full name)
__(Rm.#) __(name of) House Office Building
United States House of Representatives
Washington, DC 20515
Dear Representative:

Meeting with Elected Officials

To meet in person with an elected official, make an appointment, arrive on time, and come prepared. Understand the pros and cons of the issue you are bringing to the person's attention. Be a constructive opponent. Argue for your position and be prepared with additional information and alternative suggestions. Still, be realistic. What you want may not be possible or may not be likely at the present time. Always be helpful. Show how your issue benefits the official's constituents and thus the representative.

The American Association of Critical-Care Nurses (AACN) suggests pointers for working with public officials (American Association of Critical-Care Nurses, 2010). In addition, both the AACN and the American Nurses Association (ANA) have legislative and government information for nurses. (See links to these organizations in the Web Resources at the end of this chapter.)

Savvy nurses can use their considerable political skills to improve patient care in individual institutions, help organizations survive and thrive, and enhance nursing's image in the public arena. The political clout of this nation's more than 3 million nurses—the largest group of professionals in health care—is almost inconceivable.

Imagine what could change if nursing took advantage of this incredible potential!

What You Know Now

You have learned that politics is the ability to acquire resources to achieve your goals. You understand that policies exist in all organizations and that they emerge from the political activities of their members and leaders. You have learned the steps in political action, and you understand that behind-the-scenes work is essential to meet your goals. You know that nurses can influence both politics and policies.

You are prepared to be political.

Tools for Using Politics

1. Select people you consider to be politically savvy. Pay attention to their style of interacting with others. Adapt some of their behaviors, if appropriate, to your interactive skills.
2. Use the steps in political action to promote your ideas.
3. Learn to use behind-the-scenes strategies to support or oppose proposals.
4. Confront a person who goes behind your back to oppose you. Don't let the person get away with this tactic.
5. Monitor issues concerning health care and nursing and follow up with officials if appropriate.

Learning Activities

1. Attend a policy meeting, such as the state board of nursing, your city planning council, or a neighborhood association. Observe those who are successful in convincing others to support their goals. What did they do or not do to be successful?

2. Interview a person you consider to be influential. Ask the person to describe the process he or she uses to achieve goals. Listen for strategies that involve before and after the meeting activities as described in the chapter. If you know the person well enough, ask about behind-the-scenes efforts.
3. Prepare a proposal for a hypothetical policy change. Mentally follow the steps of political action, noting opposing opinions and how you might overcome them. Share your experiences with another person or a class.

References

American Association of Critical Care Nurses. (2010). Advocacy 101: Golden rules for those who work with public officials. Retrieved October 22, 2010, from http://www.aacn.org/wd/practice/content/publicpolicy/goldenrules.pcms?pid=1&mid=2874&menu=Community

Beall, F. (2007). Overview and summary: Power to influence patient care: Who holds the keys? *Online Journal of Issues in Nursing, 12*(1). Retrieved October 22, 2010, from http://www.nursingworld.org/MainMenuCategories/ANAMarketplace/ANAPeriodicals/OJIN/TableofContents/Volume122007/No1Jan07/tpc32ntr16088.aspx

Green, C. G., & Chaney, L. H. (2006). The game of office politics. *Supervision, 67*(8), 3–6.

Mason, D. J., Leavitt, J. K., & Chaffee, M. W. (2011). *Policy and politics in nursing and health care* (6th ed.). Philadelphia: W. B. Saunders.

Web Resources

American Association of Critical-Care Nurses, http://www.aacn.org
American Nurses Association, http://www.nursingworld.org
National Conference of State Legislatures, http://www.ncsl.org
RN Activist Kit, http://www.nursingworld.org/gova
United States House of Representatives, http://www.house.gov
United States Senate, http://www.senate.gov

CASE STUDY

In-House Political Action

As a nurse on the fourth floor of County General Rehabilitation Hospital, Ebony worked with her peers to care for patients with spinal cord injuries. The patients required frequent lifting, turning, and physical assistance in completing life care tasks. Although the nurses loved taking care of these special patients, this work was physically challenging, and staff members often suffered from back injuries and strained muscles.

Ebony met with her colleagues to brainstorm ways to improve their workplace. Doubling the number of staff would help. So might new lift equipment or assistive devices. They considered these two options.

Next, they explored the cost of equipment and the expense to train staff to use it. They identified equipment vendors. They found out how many back injuries staff had reported in the last year. In addition, they researched the national average cost of a workplace back injury and the expense of nursing turnover to an organization.

After two months, Ebony and her peers agreed on their priority: new lift equipment. They prepared a report to present to their nursing director. At the meeting, Ebony shared that they were all passionate about their work, but that they were concerned about injuries that had occurred and could occur in the future. She reported how many injuries had been reported and the national average cost of injuries and staff turnover in comparison to how much lift equipment and training for staff would cost.

"I'm impressed," the director said. "This is a well-thought plan you've prepared."

As a result, the nursing director contacted two vendors that the group had identified and scheduled a trial of the lift equipment. Ebony and her peers were proud of the work they had done to advocate for an important change in their workplace conditions.

PART

II

Using Influence

7

Setting Goals and Making Things Happen

We are all time travelers on a journey into the future.

EDWARD CORNISH, PAST PRESIDENT, WORLD FUTURE SOCIETY

In this chapter, you will learn:

- How to create a vision of your future
- How to set realistic goals
- How to decide on actions to meet your goals
- How to take advantage of opportunities
- How to select activities that further your goals

A VISION FOR YOUR FUTURE

The future is always uncertain, which leads many people to believe they cannot do anything about it. Not so. The future is shaped by human decisions and actions, including our own. What any one person cannot do is control the future. Nonetheless, we are affecting the future by what we do or fail to do today.

The future seems like something over which we have so little control that it isn't realistic to plan for it. Wait to see what happens, try to handle the circumstances, and hope for the best is as much planning as most people do. But futurists suggest a better way to prepare for the future.

Ways to Look at the Future

Previous work by Hancock and Bezold (1994) suggests that the future can be examined from several perspectives. The *possible* future includes a wide range of possibilities and encompasses everything that might happen. The possible future includes *wildcards*, events that have a low likelihood of occurring but have a high impact if they do, such as uprisings in the middle East, the 9/11 attacks, or the 2011 earthquake and tsunami in Japan. Although we need to be able to deal with wildcard incidents when they occur, our time is better spent focusing on events that are more likely to happen.

The *probable* future is based on what is happening now and our guesses about what will follow. The future is seen as an extension of today's trends. Often, this future is the one that won't happen and the one we don't want. If the census in your hospital is dropping 5 percent per year, for example, you could predict that eventually you would have no patients. That is unlikely because few hospitals would remain open until every last patient left.

The *preferable* future is what we want to have happen (Cornish, 2004). The preferable future uses a strategy of envisioning a future that does not yet exist and taking action to create it. Conceiving of a preferred future is a challenging, creative activity that organizations use to plan their business strategies. Individuals can use them, too.

Visioning is the process of imagining our preferred future and deciding on the steps to make that future happen. The vision is not the goal. It is an image of a possibility. Much can and will change to alter that image, but without it, we're unlikely to take any action toward achieving it.

For the Novice Nurse

You know about goals. You set one when you decided to become a nurse and another if you chose a partner or had a child. You chose still another if you bought a home, purchased a car, or took a yoga class. In each case, you decided upon a goal and began the process of achieving it. And then you did. Now you have the opportunity to use those goal-setting skills in your professional life. This chapter shows you how.

Envisioning Your Goals

Nurses are used to setting goals, but typically these are in terms of patient outcomes, not to envision our own future. Setting goals also is not like making New Year's resolutions, which are generally unrealistic; few survive the month of January. Envisioning goals focuses on the positives and your vision of the preferred future (Scarlett, 2010).

Several problems, however, interfere with goal setting. Identifying goals does not occur in a vacuum. It involves considering everything about you, including your past experiences, your relationships, and your environment.

Also, there are so many options that it is difficult to make a choice. Should you accept the nurse manager's job or wait to see if you are offered the position at another hospital where you applied? Would you rather have the extra money that the new job includes or more time to do things you enjoy?

Even once you've decided on a goal (e.g., go to graduate school), other opportunities can emerge (e.g., you're offered a new job that will make it difficult to attend class). Making choices is a constant. Get used to it.

In addition, the world around you keeps changing. The moment you accept the manager job, you learn that the hospital is to be sold to a for-profit health care conglomerate and your clinical area is to be combined with another hospital's. It is no wonder people often think the future is out of their control.

Finally, there are the other people in our lives to consider. Our spouse or significant other, children, parents, and friends all are essential to our life and our well-being. Pleasing all of them is not possible or appropriate. Nevertheless, their wishes and decisions bear on decisions we make and ours on them.

For the purposes of planning, though, think about what you would like to have happen in your future without regard to your significant others. Imagine all the possibilities (Borgatti, 2007). This is not an exercise that can be done instantaneously; it requires thinking, mulling over, and what people who study creativity call "time for incubation."

Matching Your Goals with Reality

Now come back to the present. Ask yourself the questions listed in Table 7-1. Also consider possible external changes that might constrain or support your goal. An increase in births, for example, might encourage you to follow your dream of becoming a nurse midwife. Be careful, though, not to fall into the trap of thinking only of the probable future. If you dream of becoming a nurse midwife, but you learn that there are only a few positions available in your area, you might decide to pursue your dream anyway. Someone will be hired for those positions, and it might be you.

Assess yourself honestly, but not too critically. Can you correct or accommodate weaknesses that might prevent you from achieving your goal? Can you build on your strengths?

TABLE 7-1 Questions to Ask about Setting Goals
What external reality could prevent you from realizing your goal?
What strengths can help you meet your goal?
Do any other goals interfere with meeting this goal?
Is there an opportunity for you to pursue this goal?
Do you want to do what it takes to achieve this goal?
Are you willing to try to correct your weaknesses to meet the goal?
Is this goal a good fit for you?

In order to achieve your goal, you may need to obtain a graduate degree, complete a certificate program, or gain experience working in a clinical area. Sometimes, those opportunities are not available in your local region or via online courses. Are you willing and able to move to acquire the education and experience you need?

Finally, decide whether this goal is right for you. No one knows you better than you know yourself. An experienced ICU nurse enrolled in a nurse practitioner program that touted the increased autonomy and income their graduates enjoyed. She left after a few weeks, returning to the ICU. "I got tired of feeling people's bellies and looking at well people," she said. "I need more action." She discovered what wasn't right for her.

Picture yourself having achieved your goal ("Successful goal setting," 2007). This step is like trying on a new style of clothes. At first, they feel strange. They are different from what you are used to wearing. Try "wearing" your goal for a while. See if the fit is good enough for you to keep it. Try your idea out on people you trust. They may point out aspects you had not considered. Just realize that no one else can make your decision for you.

Maybe this goal isn't right for you at this time. Sometimes, waiting is the best decision. Again, you must decide.

Balancing your goals with your desires, talents, situation, and opportunities is not an easy task but is one that pays big dividends for your future.

It's worth it.

Decide on Your Time Frame

Whether we realize it or not, we are constantly setting goals. A to-do list is an example of a short-term goal. Time pressure makes these activities fairly easy to discover for both work and home.

Most of us have many years in a career, and some of us will have more than one occupation. If you are 22 when you graduate from college today, you will have nearly 50 years until you are eligible for Social Security. The bulk of your life will be spent working. You want it to be the best you can make it, so it pays to plan for it.

The careers of parents—especially women—are often erratic, alternating time in and time out of the workforce as the demands of childrearing, education, and their spouse's work fluctuate. Nurses, like people employed in other fields, work varying flex-time, part-time, and full-time schedules according to their and their employer's needs. Such erratic arrangements suggest that planning is useless. Therein lies the importance of visioning flexible goals that you can adapt to your own circumstances and opportunities that emerge.

> A nurse met with the advisor in a baccalaureate program designed for RNs. After talking about the requirements of the program, the classes she needed and her own schedule, they concluded that it would take the nurse five years to complete the program by taking one course a semester. The RN looked discouraged. The advisor asked her what was wrong.

> "In five years I'll be 35 if I enroll in this program," she said. The advisor smiled. "Yes, and you'll be 35 in five years if you don't."

Imagine yourself one year from now, creating in your mind the life you most desire. What are you doing? What have you done over the course of the past year? The answers to those two questions suggest a one-year goal and the actions needed to accomplish it.

Now imagine what you are doing in five years, then ten years. Use the same strategy to create plans to meet your longer-term goals.

What will you be doing right before you retire? Will you be satisfied with what you've done? What do you wish you had done? That is your long-term goal. It consists of many short-term goals over the course of your career.

What if, you ask, everything doesn't work out as I've imagined it? Actually, it probably won't—regardless of how carefully you plan. Adjustments must be made continually.

The map is not the journey. Just as a map helps guide us toward a destination, so our plan serves as a guide to help us meet our goal. Detours occur or new scenery beckons, altering our route, but the destination remains the same. Keep it flexible. Allow for unplanned events, such as illness, pregnancy, or your hospital closing. Plan for contingencies, but keep your eye on your vision.

Your attitude is the most important characteristic you can bring to goal setting. Knowing that you deserve it and being willing to do whatever it takes to achieve it are essential.

Have courage. Ignore naysayers. It's not their goal; it's yours.

MAKING IT HAPPEN

Choosing the Organization

The first step for most of us after graduation is to decide where to go to work. (You will learn more about obtaining your first job in Chapter 13.) The determining factor in most cases is salary.

> A faculty member asked her students, who were due to graduate in a few weeks, if they had jobs (most did) and how they decided on the job they accepted. Starting salary, most said, citing minimal differences among hospitals.
>
> The savvy faculty member shook her head. "That's not the best reason," she said, going on to explain how they should use every job to prepare them for their next one or to further their career, such as giving them experience in a specific clinical area.
>
> This instructor knew the way to make goals happen.

Finding the organization that fits you is more difficult than it sounds. Most of us assume that one hospital or one clinic is much like another. Just attending class should tell you that such is not the case.

Every group or organization develops a culture based on its purpose, structure, and the interactions of its members. These vary widely and are sustained even when the purpose, structure, or members change, much like an ethnic culture remains more or less the same for generations. Many an executive has thought to change an institution's culture only to learn that instead, he or she had to change or leave the organization.

This is not to say, however, that each individual has no effect on the organization. In fact, each person does affect the organization, and the organization affects each person in it. Just don't expect the organization to change radically. That is why it is so important for you to discover as much as you can about the organization's culture *before* you become involved in it.

But, you ask, how can I learn about an organization's culture? Don't expect it to be on their website or in recruiting material or for it to be described outright in an interview. In fact, little will be written anywhere about its culture. Similar to influence and image, culture controls the context and frames everything that happens, whether it concerns an individual or an organization. There are ways, however, of learning about an organization's culture.

You can glean some information from printed material. If, for example, you are interested in a graduate program and the literature you receive includes such statements as, "The student will not be admitted if … ," assume that the culture of the school is more punitive than inviting.

Interviews also offer some telling information. The manner in which you are treated (e.g., whether you are greeted warmly or kept waiting) sends a message. Taking a tour gives you an excellent opportunity to pick up atmosphere and unspoken messages and to read expressions and body language.

Best of all, use your networks of friends, colleagues, and fellow students. Anyone who has worked at the institution or on a specific unit has learned about the culture. Ask them. You might decide that although what you hear is negative for that person, it wouldn't be for you. Your colleague might say the nurses were too busy to talk; you might decide you'd enjoy the challenge of a fast-paced environment.

The rumor mill is another excellent source of information. Remember, though, that most rumors are not exactly correct. Usually, they are a slightly altered version of the truth. Also, your colleague might not assess an organization using the same criteria you would. Just use rumors and friends' opinions as pieces of information to help you decide what is right for you.

Opportunities in Professional Associations

Few people think of professional associations as career-enhancing strategies. One group, however, has made leadership development a key component of its mission. Sigma Theta Tau International's Leadership Institute is designed to prepare nursing leaders for influential positions in organizations and policy making institutions. (See the end-of-chapter Web Resources section.)

Lack of member involvement is a commonly heard complaint in most professional associations as well as among community groups. For the career-minded person, a professional organization offers valuable contacts and opportunities to develop and hone your influence-making skills. Thus, the organization gains helpers to do the work while it builds future leaders for the profession. Members receive training that they can use on their jobs and to enhance their future prospects. Both gain more influence to further their goals. Likewise, community organizations, such as Toastmasters groups, Rotary clubs, or nonprofit community agencies offer similar opportunities to make contacts and learn leadership skills. Take advantage of ones that draw your interest and can use your skills.

Choosing a professional association is just as important as deciding on a paid position. You need to learn all you can about the organization's mission, its manner of operating, and its culture before deciding whether it is the right one for you. Because organizations usually need help, your interest may encourage someone to invite your participation. However, be sure that this is the right organization for you at this time.

Myriad organizations exist and clamor for our time. Specialty organizations designed to meet specific needs of nurses in clinical areas of practice, such as the AACN, as well as organizations for all registered nurses, such as the American Nurses Association, compete with each other for our allegiance, our time, and our money. Membership can be maintained in several organizations, and our involvement in each may vary over the course of our careers.

After you've done your homework about the organizations and decided that the goals of one fit with yours, it's time to let association leaders know about your interest. Attend meetings of the group, such as your local chapter of Sigma Theta Tau International or state nurses' association. Let people know informally that you're interested in becoming involved. Also, you can contact a few key people in the organization directly and let them know that you are interested in helping them meet their goals. You will undoubtedly be warmly welcomed. Don't push, though. The leader may not be able to think of how to involve you immediately. You don't need to know the details. Leave it up to them.

Follow up all contacts with a brief note, thanking them for their time and again expressing your interest. If, after a while, no one has responded to your invitation, let it go and find somewhere else to offer your services. Although the lack of response may just indicate that the person to whom you spoke lacked the skills to take advantage of your offer, you don't want to be part of an ineffective organization. Be sure to talk to more than one person to avoid this result.

Selling Yourself

You know something about the organization, either for a paid position or as a volunteer, and how your interest, talent, and skills fit with the organization's goals. Now it's time to sell yourself. No one can do it as well as you can.

Be as specific as possible. If the job calls for someone who has experience with a newly available patient monitoring device and you have used it, tell the interviewer about this experience. Emphasize your strengths; don't mention your weaknesses. If asked, however, have some characteristic in mind that you can use as an example of a weakness. Your impatience may be annoying to your family, but an employer might view it positively. It means you are motivated to get the work done.

Never, never lie. Even if you are never caught, you will spend your entire career looking over your shoulder and wondering if anyone has found out that you didn't finish the graduate program you listed on your résumé. There is no need, however, to point out that you didn't finish the program; just don't say you did. Often, events that we think will stand out on a résumé or in an interview are unimportant to a potential employer.

Follow up your interview with a brief note, just as you would to indicate interest in a professional association. For a job, though, if you haven't heard in a week or so, you can send a brief e-mail or leave a short phone message to indicate that you are still interested in the position. Don't press. Be courteous, pleasant, and businesslike.

Saying No

Sometimes we decide to decline offers for jobs, admission to educational programs, or voluntary positions in organizations—even positions we would like to have. The tendency is to agree because the work is something we would enjoy or would help us, and—let's admit it—it's flattering to be asked. Take time, though, to decide whether this opportunity is right for you at this time.

> A well-known nurse leader reluctantly turned down the very flattering offer to be nominated as president of a major nursing organization. She had just accepted a position on another organization's board and was recovering from a lengthy illness. She believed in the organization's mission and knew she could contribute to its future. In fact, she was excited about the possibilities that serving as president would offer her and the organization. She also knew that if she declined, she might not have another chance at the position. Nonetheless, she knew herself well enough that she knew the time wasn't right.
>
> Surprisingly, two years later she received a call. Would she be a candidate this time? She was elected and served as the organization's president during an important time in the expansion of the association.

We don't always make perfect decisions for ourselves or an organization. We accept a job and discover later that it was wrong for us. We learned something. We learn, too, when something we wanted doesn't work out. Often we find out later that not getting the job turned out to be the best decision for us, even though we couldn't see this fact at the time. That's life. Just keep honing your skills to assess yourself and collect the information you need to make decisions. It's the best anyone can do.

Whether an offer comes from a potential employer or a professional association, let the representative know that you appreciate the offer and that you hope they will keep you in mind in the future. Be sure to keep the door open and your relationship cordial.

WHEN THE GOING GETS TOUGH

Making plans is relatively easy when things go our way. The nursing shortage, the availability of jobs, well-developed clinical skills, and a positive reputation in your area widen your choices: an enviable position. When things go wrong, however, it's more difficult. Cutbacks, an easing of the shortage, your hospital is sold, your job disappears, you get pregnant, your spouse gets transferred, the children are ill, or your parents need help: all events like these can interfere with the best-laid plans. The axiom "When the going gets tough, the tough get going" is never truer then. Adversity separates the strong from the weak.

Accepting the Risk

High goals and high risks go together. Successful people take a lot of risks, and they have failures. People who take few risks have failures, but because they so seldom risk, the failures are more apparent. Fear and pain could occur with success as well as failure. The key is how you use a failure to learn what you would do in the future.

Making a mistake is not fatal. It's just a mistake.

Planning for the Rest of Your Life

The first day of a new job is the time to think about your next one (Cardillo, 2008). Build a network both inside the organization and among colleagues elsewhere. Listen for opportunities; if you might be interested, let people know you'd like to talk more about the possibilities. Always be looking. Just don't be obvious about it.

Jobs have a predictable cycle. In the beginning is the honeymoon period. You're the center of attention, forgiven much, and excited to be embarking on a new path. Next comes the period of building your skills, learning about the organization, and enjoying your role in its success. The maintenance period evolves next. Now you know the work and the people, and not much new occurs. Finally, you're only going through the motions and watching the clock until it's time to go home. It's time to leave.

The same cycle occurs in voluntary positions. That's the reason for term limits for board and committee members. Too long in one position makes anyone redundant. And it doesn't allow for other members to become involved, infusing the organization with new views and ideas.

No matter how committed you are, how much you have done for the organization, or how much people there like you, eventually you will run out of ideas and get tired and things will go wrong. It happens to everyone. If you wait to leave until then, you will be remembered for the last things that happened, not the first when you did so well.

Leaving when you're on top benefits you and the organization. You've given them your very best ideas, energy, and commitment. You will be remembered for your contributions more than your mistakes. Keep your memories—both good and not-so-good—and learn to know when it's time to move on, and do it.

Leaving the Organization

Change is difficult for everyone; leaving a job is especially difficult. You have made friends, some of whom you'll lose contact with over time, no matter how much you vow not to. Some will tell you horror stories about what will happen with the void your absence will bring. They are wrong. Removing a cup of water from a bucket shows you what happens when a void is created. Someone or something fills it. So it is with organizations. Your leaving gives someone else a chance, whose leaving gives another person an opportunity, and so on.

What You Know Now

You have learned three ways to look at the future: the possible, the probable, and the preferable. You know that visioning a preferred future is a complex, interrelated process that occurs in the context of our relationships, our environments, and our personalities. You learned that goals change and evolve as circumstances in our lives change and that successful people learn to modify their goals while keeping an eye on their vision. You have learned how to assess an organization for your involvement and that these criteria apply to employment opportunities as well as participation in a professional organization. You have learned how to sell yourself and to say no when that is appropriate. Finally, you have accepted the risks, you know that with opportunities come chances for failure, and you have learned strategies for leaving an organization.

You're on your way to fulfilling your vision of your future!

Tools for Setting and Meeting Goals

1. If the present circumstances continue, what is your probable future? What would be your preferable future?
2. Watch successful people to see what they are doing that might help them meet their goals.
3. Pay attention to possible future opportunities and try to learn as much as you can about them.

4. Imagine your dream. It can be a job or a position in an organization as a leader or a follower. Think big. See what happens.

Learning Activities

1. Write down your one-year goals. Include professional as well as personal goals. List the action steps necessary to meet your goals. Review your progress monthly and adjust goals or time frames as needed.
2. Using the concepts presented in the chapter, what do you think your probable future is? What is your preferred future? Think about how you can create your preferred future.
3. If you could do anything in the world you wanted to, what would you choose? Think of ways you could do that or something similar. Share your ideas with a friend or classmate. See if you can help each other think of ways that might lead toward the futures that each of you wants.

References

Borgatti, J. C. (2007). Plan a career, not just a job. *American Nurse Today, 2*(4). Retrieved November 5, 2010, from http://www.americannursetoday.com/article.aspx?id=6204&fid=6182

Cardillo, D. W. (2008). *The ultimate career guide for nurses.* Falls Church, VA: Gannett Healthcare Group.

Cornish, E. (2004). *Futuring: The exploration of the future.* Bethesda, MD: World Future Society.

Hancock, T., & Bezold, C. (1994). Possible futures; preferable futures. *Healthcare Forum, 36*(3), 23–29.

Scarlett, G. (2010). Using goals to grow in nursing. *Ezinearticles.com.* Retrieved November 5, 2010, from http://ezinearticles.com/?Using-Goals-to-Grow-in-Nursing&id=2127751

Successful goal setting. (2007, March 22). *NursingTimes.net.* Retrieved November 5, 2010, from http://www.nursingtimes.net/nursing-practice-clinical-research/successful-goal-setting/201212.article

Web Resources

Sigma Theta Tau International Leadership Institute, http://www.nursingsociety.org/LEADERSHIPINSTITUTE/pages/default.aspx

Sullivan, E. J. Brick by brick. *Journal of Professional Nursing, 17*(2), http://www.eleanorsullivan.com/pdf/brick.pdf

Manktelow, J., & Fowler, K. Personal goal setting, http://www.topachievement.com/articles/personalgoalsetting.html

Then, J. Goal setting: The key to success, http://ezinearticles.com/?Goal-Setting---The-Key-to-Success&id=304851

Lim, S. Top 5 secrets to successful smart goal setting, http://ezinearticles.com/?Top-5-Secrets-to-Successful-Smart-Goal-Setting&id=1334937

CASE STUDY

Setting and Meeting Goals

Lana enjoyed taking care of acutely ill patients on the cardiology step-down unit where she had worked for four years. When Lana met with her manager, Eloise, for her annual performance appraisal, she received an exemplary review. "What's your goal for next year?" Eloise asked.

Lana didn't know. "Go home and think about what you might want to accomplish," Eloise told her. "It should be something important to you."

Lana had been thinking about becoming an ICU nurse. This year, she decided, she'd focus on that goal. She wanted to build on the skills she had developed with cardiology patients and to begin taking care of more complex, critically ill patients.

"What do I need to be successful?" Lana asked herself.

She made a list. First, she updated her résumé to reflect her goal to work in an ICU. She listed her strengths. They were: dependable, willing to learn, and flexible in any circumstance.

She also thought about her weaknesses. She knew at times she was fearful of putting herself forward. Even when she had the correct answer to a question, she could be timid and not confident enough to speak up. She decided to focus on refining these weaknesses by intentionally choosing learning opportunities that forced her to speak out and to offer her expertise to coworkers without hesitating.

Next she shared her goal with Eloise, who was supportive. Lana asked Eloise to tell the ICU manager about Lana's work ethic and performance. In addition, Lana e-mailed the ICU manager, Anne, and asked if she could stop in to introduce herself during her next shift. Anne agreed.

At the meeting, Lana introduced herself with enthusiasm and gave Anne a copy of her updated résumé. She shared that she had been a nurse in the step-down unit for more than four years and that she was eager to expand her skills and work in an ICU.

"Watch for job postings, and I'd be happy to interview you when a position is open," Anne told her.

Five months later, Lana saw a position posted for an ICU nurse position. During these months, Lana had taken additional continuing education classes about critically ill patient care. She applied for the position and Anne interviewed her, then introduced her to staff members on the unit for a peer interview. After these interviews, Lana knew that she would like to work on this unit.

One week later, Anne called and offered her the position. Lana was so excited, and she accepted. She was proud of herself. She had made a plan to accomplish her goal and prepared herself to get the job she wanted—and she had succeeded!

8

Making Connections and Building Coalitions

Human nature is the same all over the world.

EARL OF CHESTERFIELD, 1747

In this chapter, you will learn:

- Why it is important to build a network
- What a coalition can do that you can't do alone
- When to compete and when to support
- How helping others can help you
- How to persuade others to join your coalition

HOW TO MAKE CONNECTIONS

This chapter is about relationships among people who have something in common (e.g., other nurses), who have something to share, or who are looking for something now or in the future (e.g., a job). These relationships are honest and reciprocal, although exact exchanges seldom occur—at least not at the same time. The people involved may become close personal friends, but that is not the goal of these relationships. They are designed to fit the rules, as described in Chapter 2, and to benefit both parties.

Meeting People

"It isn't who you know, it's who knows you," according to Arvin (2009). The way people get to know you—especially influential people—is by what you do. Here are some suggestions:

- Do your job well.
- Share your accomplishments appropriately.
- Attend important meetings.
- Join and participate in social media networks (e.g., Facebook, LinkedIn).
- Try to find commonalities with the people you meet in person or online.

At meetings, arrive early to have an opportunity to meet others. Sit near the front and center in meetings; avoid sitting with people you know. Introduce yourself to others, including the speakers or leaders.

Want to know how to *not* make connections at meetings? Take your personal items, find a seat, and plant yourself. Talk only to people you know. Leave as soon as the meeting is over. Avoid talking to the powerful people.

Remember the meetings before and after the meeting discussed in Chapter 6? Use both those times to connect with people you'd like to meet and—more importantly—those you want to have met you. You can do this online and in person.

For the Novice Nurse

Even if you don't realize it, you already have many people in your network. Your teachers, your classmates, nurses in clinical settings, and your coworkers are all in your network. Plus, you have friends, family members, neighbors, and people in formal organizations and informal groups. So stop right now and begin a list of people in your network. It will be longer than you expect.

Small Talk

As you learned in Chapter 1, small talk is neither small nor unimportant. Learning and using small talk is one of the most valuable skills you can develop to put you on the way to becoming influential.

Small talk is an equal sharing between two or more people. Small talk is a pleasant way to enjoy the time you are spending with others, to make connections, to share ideas and information, and to set the stage for opportunities in the future (Baber & Waymon, 2007). Small talk helps participants feel more comfortable in social situations, and it can smooth the way for immediate or future in-depth interactions. There is no downside to small talk.

Small talk involves mutual sharing, a back and forth of information and ideas. To make small talk, you can ask and answer questions, comment on the other person's statements, and ask directly for what you want. Here are some examples:

- Ask a question: "Where do you work?"
- Answer a question: "I'm a nurse doing research at St. Teresa's Hospital in intensive care."
- Comment on other person's statement: "That sounds interesting. I've done some research myself" and follow with "What are you trying to find out?"
- Ask directly for what you want: "I'm looking for a place to do my management practicum. Do you know of anyone who might be interested?"

These statements might get the conversation going, and if you stay present in the conversation (not looking around for someone else whom you might approach), you will find that they lead to additional comments, questions, and ideas. Sometimes, however, you will encounter people who don't understand the equality necessary for small talk to proceed or who don't respond to your statements or questions. They drop the proverbial ball. In that case, it's up to you to throw out another statement or question designed to elicit a response.

STRATEGIES FOR SMALL TALK. Cultivate your curiosity and a desire for discovery, focusing on the other person. Try to connect, not perform or compete, in conversational games such as one-upmanship. The purpose of small talk is to learn what you have in common, not to show how good or important you are.

Follow up with any promise you make. For example, say you meet a nurse recruiter at a local nursing association meeting and she tells you she's looking for an experienced nurse manager for their ER. You have a colleague who is just finishing a degree in management and who has been a trauma nurse. You offer to pass the nurse recruiter's card along to your colleague. You do so.

Now you have made contact with someone you didn't know and who is likely to remember you; besides, your colleague will appreciate your thinking of him or her, regardless of whether the colleague takes the position. (It's a good idea to ask for two business cards if you are planning to pass one of them on so that you can contact the other person later if needed.)

Sometimes, interactions are not as they appear. Someone's real agenda may be hidden, and may make participants feel uncomfortable. That feeling is manipulation. It is much better to make your agenda apparent and state straightforwardly that you are looking for a job, trying to find a good cardiologist for your mother, or soliciting candidates for your organization's slate of officers. Being straightforward does not mean you have to disclose anything you wouldn't want to share; it means only that you need to be clear about what you want *from that person in that situation*.

Use your body language and ways of speaking to encourage others to respond. Eye contact, tone of voice, gestures, nods, and body position can

TABLE 8-1 Using Nonverbal Cues

To encourage	To discourage
Keep eye contact longer than your partner.	Look away often, pay attention to others.
Lean toward your partner.	Lean away or step back.
Face your partner.	Turn your shoulder toward your partner.
Nod and smile appropriately.	Keep a straight face regardless of your partner's words.

Note: Some cultural variations occur in nonverbal communication.

express your interest in the other person, as well as the words you say. (You'll learn more about others' nonverbal behaviors in Chapter 11.)

Table 8-1 illustrates ways in which nonverbal cues can be used to encourage or discourage responses. However, these cues differ among cultures. For example, in some cultures, maintaining eye contact more than briefly is considered impolite. Body movement, facial expressions, and gestures are all subject to cultural connotations.

LEAVE THE CONVERSATION BUT NOT THE RELATIONSHIP. Baber and Waymon (2007) also suggest ways to exit the conversation without losing the connection to the other person and without feeling awkward. They suggest closing with statements that express your purpose for the small talk, respond to what the other person has asked of you, or promise to follow up on whatever you've learned during the conversation. Here are some examples:

- ***Focus on your agenda.*** "I want to speak to some of the officers of our organization before the meeting starts." Shake hands, add some words about how nice it was to talk with the person, and leave. Don't hang around acting like you're afraid of hurting the person's feelings by walking away. Give people credit for taking care of themselves.
- ***Take your partner with you.*** "I see my coworker just came in and you wanted to meet her." Then take your small talk partner with you.
- ***Summarize the conversation and express your appreciation.*** "I'm glad we had time to talk about our committee." Thank the person graciously and move on.
- ***Say what you will do next.*** "I'll send you the information about the graduate program you're interested in."

At times, you may need to develop skills to get away from overly talkative people in some circumstances. Interrupt politely and excuse yourself in these situations. You can add that you are hoping to talk to others at the meeting, smile, and leave. Don't linger, feeling sorry for abandoning the person.

Small talk skills can lead to future interactions and relationships. These, in turn, help you build a network.

BUILDING A NETWORK

Networking is the exchange of information and services in such a way as to create relationships (Baber & Waymon, 2007). "Networking is one of the most valuable skills a nurse can develop," says Donna Cardillo, a well-known nurse speaker and author (Ondash, 2010).

Networking is reciprocal. You help others and they help you. Your agenda is aboveboard, not hidden. Your goal should be to give more than you get. If everyone begins with that goal in mind, everyone benefits.

Social media, online discussion groups, and contact management systems have changed the landscape for building and using a network. Friends can introduce you to someone whose interests parallel yours through social media sites. You can discover like-minded people in online discussion groups on Yahoo, Facebook, or LinkedIn. (See more on using social media in the section "Expanding Your Network" later in this chapter.)

Each encounter offers an opportunity to add someone to your network and for other people to add you to theirs. Casual meetings, organized events, and online interactions offer opportunities for getting to know others. Sometimes we don't know a way in which another person can help us or vice versa. No matter. Be aware that future possibilities might emerge and treat each person accordingly. Sometimes, a simple act of kindness can result in long-term benefits.

> An experienced nurse researcher agreed to meet with a nurse acquaintance who was contemplating graduate school. On the way to their lunch appointment, however, the potential student had a minor accident. Calling her higher-level colleague from the ER, she explained that although she wasn't seriously injured, she'd have to miss their appointment. The experienced researcher asked where her car was. Towed to the body shop, explained the nurse.
>
> The experienced researcher offered to pick up the nurse, whom she only knew from a brief conversation, and drive her home, going a long way out of her way. This kindness was never forgotten by the student who, beyond writing her a personal, hand-written thank you, told the story often to other people.

This example shows how each time we encounter another person, we have an opportunity to benefit both of us. Remember, you're building reciprocal relationships; giving is more important than getting.

Your Network

Your professional work and personal life offer many opportunities for building a network. (See Table 8-2.) Those closest to you are your first-level network and those who are more distant become your second- and third-level networks. Of course, many people overlap levels and become closer or more distant at different times.

TABLE 8-2 Your Networks

Professional	Personal
First Level	**First Level**
Immediate workgroup	Immediate family
Peers in similar positions at your institution	Close friends
Professional colleagues in other disciplines	
Subordinates	
Superiors	
Current instructors	
Second Level	**Second Level**
Top-level administrator at your institution	Relatives
Other staff members	Neighbors
Nurses at other institutions	Business acquaintances
Classmates and former classmates	Other acquaintances
Members of professional associations	
Former instructors	
Acquaintances at work	
Third Level	**Third Level**
Associate deans and dean(s) of your school(s)	Religious association leaders
Chairs of your institutions' boards (university/hospital)	Local business owners
State and federal legislators and officials	Local officials
Officers in professional associations	Other school, neighborhood, and local leaders
People you meet at conventions and events	

Your closest colleagues at work form your initial network. Even if you leave the job or they do, you can find ways to still include them in your network. Peers at work (e.g., nurses in similar positions), professionals in other disciplines (e.g., physicians, social workers, physical therapists), your subordinates and superiors (because you never know when your positions might be reversed), other staff members (e.g., clerks, admitting staff), classmates and former classmates, members of professional associations, and others you may meet in your work world (e.g., pharmaceutical salespeople) form your network. You can likely think of others. More distant are leaders of schools you've attended, legislators, and officers of your professional associations.

Your immediate family and close friends make up the nucleus of your personal network. Relatives, neighbors, and business acquaintances form the next level of your network. Leaders of associations (e.g., your child's parent-teacher organization) and local officials (e.g., police department) are farther removed.

Expanding Your Network

IN PERSON. Every meeting, every chance encounter, and every introduction offers an opportunity to build your network. That said, use your judgment about the appropriateness of adding someone to your network. Add those you think you can help, those who might help you, and those with whom you have a common interest. That list will include many people.

Attending professional association meetings is an excellent way to network. The leaders in your profession are often the leaders in the organization, and the members who aspire to be leaders attend meetings. "Stay with the winners" is a business adage that you should heed.

You can have your choice among organizations so that you can find one that meets your needs. Your clinical specialty group might be right for you. You may prefer your state nurses' association or your local chapter of Sigma Theta Tau International. As stated in previous chapters, becoming involved with your professional association is one of the best ways to build your leadership skills, learn about important issues in the profession, and meet people who can further your career.

Use meetings at your workplace and your school, if you are a student, to learn and to meet other interested people as well as the speakers and leaders. Use the advice on small talk and make a note of people you meet.

ONLINE. Finding people with common interests is easier than ever online. You can find blogs and discussion groups on every topic imaginable. Explore groups interested in nursing, health care, career building, cabinet making, or whatever interests you. If someone has an interest similar to yours and you have a reason to do so, contact the person offline. When you post updates on Facebook or LinkedIn, they automatically arrive on your contacts' pages. Contact management systems such as iContact enable you to easily and simultaneously contact people on your network.

Join and participate in groups and blogs. Don't be just a lurker, only culling information helpful to you. Participate in the discussion, make comments, offer suggestions, and ask questions. Of course, do so appropriately and politely. Also, be certain that you have information to add; don't just inject comments to be noticed. Those who do so repeatedly are not only annoying; serious participants also tend to overlook their comments after a time.

Keeping Track of Your Network

To keep track of your network, you can use a contact management system (e.g., Constant Contact®, an app on your phone, a computer database, or daily planner). Keep notes to remind you of when and where you met, any information about the person that might be useful in the future, and ways you might help each other.

USING YOUR NETWORK

Once you have decided to develop a network and begun to build it, you are ready to use your network. The first step is staying connected. Attending professional meetings is one way to do so; seeing you there helps others keep you in mind. This is known as "face time," and every successful person knows to use it.

You meet someone at a conference or meeting and exchange phone numbers and e-mail addresses. A new acquaintance is likely to be on Facebook or LinkedIn or may have a blog. You can use e-mail or text messaging to contact him or her. Send a brief email or text to say how much you enjoyed meeting the new acquaintance and that you hope to keep in touch.

Later, if you see something online or in a professional publication that you think might interest your new contact, you can send a brief message with a link to the site or mail a copy with a short note from you. You might hear, for example, about an opening in your cardiac cath lab and know someone who might be interested. You pass the information along to your contact and offer to submit his or her name to your human resource department.

Some influential people set a goal to contact at least one person on their network each week. That is a laudable goal that you might find useful. If you can't manage that much time to maintain your network, just try to be alert to ways you can contact colleagues and take advantage of those opportunities.

Another way to use your network is for paying and collecting debts. Remember the quid pro quo discussed in Chapter 2? Anyone to whom you owe a debt or who owes you should be included in your network.

When someone whom you owe contacts you, try your best to respond. If you cannot return the favor, try to suggest someone else who can. If nothing else, be sure to tell the person that you are willing to help in the future. You've shown that you're savvy enough to know that you still owe the favor and that you're willing to do it.

When you need a favor, think about someone you can help. If the person owes you, contact the person, remind him or her of the past event, and ask your favor. You don't need to be aggressive about your reminder. Just a few words, such as, "I'm glad your new job is working out and that I was able to give you a reference for it" is enough to bring the event into mind. If the person is unable to help, possibly he or she can suggest someone else who can. If, however, the person refuses to help, be polite, end the conversation, and make a mental note about the conversation. If that person asks you for a favor in the future, you may decide to refuse. He or she isn't playing fair.

COMPETING AND SUPPORTING

When to Compete

Competing is fine—and necessary at times—but it needn't ruin a relationship. To compete but continue a relationship, you must compete fairly.

Remember the discussion about people who tell you they are supporting you but go behind your back and tell others they can't support you? Don't play a dirty trick like that. Competition should be aboveboard; if you cannot support someone, you should tell the person why. Don't go behind his or her back and do the opposite of what you've promised.

What if you're competing with a friend—for a job, maybe, or running for president of an association? Nothing's wrong with that, but be aware that such competition may interfere, at least for a time, in your relationship. You simply will not be able to be open with your friend about your strategies for winning the job or the election. You can, however, avoid such a discussion for the time being. If both people genuinely want to continue the relationship, they may be able to maintain their friendship much as it was before once a decision is made. Be aware, though, that some people will find that strategy difficult and the relationship may diminish for a time.

The competition ends when a decision is made, the ballots are counted, or the job offer accepted. When the competition's over, the game's over. Don't hold a grudge, refuse to speak to the person, or bad-mouth the person or group to others. Your relationship goes on. Remember the bear hunt? You will live to hunt again, and you may need your colleague then. Don't give up the relationship—regardless of who wins.

When to Support

Inevitably, you will be asked to support another person or group in whatever they hope to achieve. When the benefit to you is apparent and there is no disadvantage to you, your decision is easy. If you will receive something in exchange without harm to you, the decision to support is also simple. Not only will you benefit immediately in these situations, but you will garner the good will of those you are supporting.

Try to think through all the ramifications of supporting another's project:

- What are possible outcomes?
- Is the project likely to be successful?
- Can anything go wrong?
- Are other people and groups supporting the project, or are there others who have refused to support it?
- Are there any reasons why you should not support the project? What might you gain by supporting it?

If your answers convince you that the benefits outweigh the disadvantages, go ahead and support the project. Remember that you may reap a benefit in the future from the debt owed to you.

HOW TO SUPPORT. Throughout your career, you are likely to be asked for support in myriad ways, from a simple endorsement of a project being discussed in a committee meeting to committing your organization's funds for a grant proposal. Once you've decided that the project is worthy and that you are able to support it, you must decide how to support it. Sometimes, you will be able to lend the support asked. At other times, you will want to support the project but be unable to give what is asked.

Let's say, for example, that your organization has been asked to endorse a community project designed to recruit students to nursing. You are chair of the committee charged with making a recommendation to the administration. Your committee is in favor of the request, but they are reluctant to recommend the level of financial commitment that has been requested. You decide to recommend a lower level of funding while emphasizing the benefit that the project will bring to your institution.

WHEN YOU CANNOT SUPPORT. Sometimes, you will have no choice about supporting another's project. Your job or your position may dictate your response. Let's say, for example, that your institution is planning to add an outreach ambulatory care unit in a growing suburb. They are, however, keeping that information quiet until they have the approvals and resources they need. In the meantime, a colleague from another institution calls you and asks for your support for establishing a nurse-managed clinic in the same area. She wants you to write a letter to the local school of nursing, where you sit on the alumni board, encouraging the school to participate. What should you do?

Here's one way to handle this difficult request: tell your colleague that you are unable to support her request because it may conflict with your responsibilities. Apologize and wish her well. Don't explain or give details. You may be violating your responsibility to your employer if you do. This way you've been honest without betraying your employer's confidence.

Let's make this situation even more complicated. What if she asks you not to tell anyone about her plans? Should you tell your employer? In general, the answer is yes, but you must tell her that you cannot keep what she told you in confidence. "If you tell me, you tell my organization," is a possible response. At least now she knows you are honest with her even if she doesn't like the answer. She also knows that she can trust you to be forthright in the future.

These are not easy requests to handle. As with other ethical questions, the answers are not clearly right or wrong but are complicated by circumstances and competing points of view. The best you can do is to think them through, consider the pros and cons and competing loyalties, and do your best.

Staying Neutral

Sometimes you will want or need to stay neutral. This is not an easy position to maintain because opposing parties may all be trying to get your support. A political battle is a good example. You may be solicited by both candidates for mayor of your town, for example, each wanting your vote and possibly your money. You have probably found out how difficult it is to talk to friends about your political beliefs when you have opposing views. Even staying out of such hot-button discussions requires tact and determination. Keeping quiet and refusing to respond to challenges may be the only way to continue relationships in the face of pressure.

BUILDING A COALITION

The Purpose of a Coalition

A coalition is an alliance of people or groups with similar goals who join together to achieve their objectives. Coalitions may be formed for any number of purposes, and various entities constituting the coalition may have different—though complementary—goals. A coalition may be proactive, initiating activities, or reactive, preventing actions by other groups.

The coalition may be a loose collection of people that come together briefly (e.g., a task force) or may be more formally established and long lasting, such as a standing committee. Regardless, a coalition can achieve what no one individual or group can achieve on its own.

The American Nurses Association (ANA), as a federation of state nurses associations, is a formal coalition. ANA, in turn, belongs to other coalitions, such as the Tri-Council of Nursing Organizations that consists of representatives from ANA, the American Association of Colleges of Nursing, the National League for Nursing, and the American Organization of Nurse Executives. In addition, the representatives from various nursing organizations often join together to achieve a specific, time-limited goal, such as promoting nurses for positions on federal advisory boards. This is an example of an ad hoc, issue-oriented coalition.

Proactive coalitions are established to create or change existing conditions. The creation of the National Institute of Nursing Research within the National Institutes of Health (NIH), as reported in Chapter 6, is an example. In this case, numerous nursing organizations formed a coalition that targeted members of Congress and NIH directors and continued their lobbying until they were successful.

Reactive coalitions are formed to thwart a specific threat (e.g., proposed change in a nursing practice act to restrict the scope of practice). These may be short-lived efforts involving rapid and concerted responses to potential problems. Various nursing groups within the state, for example, might form a coalition to lobby state legislators to vote against changing the nursing practice act, citing the reduced availability of nursing care to the legislators' constituents.

Both proactive and reactive coalitions, by their very nature, could produce conflict. Challenging the power structure of institutions, organizations, or bureaucracies requires commitment and fortitude. That is why members need to be involved and resolute. It is much easier to stand firm against opposition when you stand together.

Sometimes coalitions are formed without a specific agenda in mind. Members of these coalitions expect that they will need each others' support in the future and that there likely will be opportunities when their mutual support will benefit all of them. By forming a coalition ahead of time, groups can discover common goals and interests, develop trust, and be prepared to move rapidly in the face of threats or to achieve mutual goals.

Two conditions increase the likelihood that a coalition will be successful. First, the structure of the coalition must encourage the participation of all members. Those who will be most affected must be involved and committed.

Second, the process of deliberation and decision making must take into account the needs and desires of all members, even if everyone's goals cannot be accomplished. All members must have an opportunity to explain their goals, and the group must work collectively and collaboratively to meet the needs of as many of the members' goals as possible.

The work of the coalition, however, should not be compromised or diluted just so that everyone's goals can be included. A balance must be struck between meeting the goal of the coalition and meeting individual members' goals. The important point is that each member has an opportunity to be heard and that all members' wishes are considered.

Forming a Coalition

The first step in forming a coalition is to identify the issue or problem (see Box 8-1). Often the issue or problem emerges from an external threat, such as the threatened restrictions on nursing practice mentioned previously. Other times, one or more individuals or groups recognize an opportunity and set about to enlighten potential partners.

The second step is to identify groups or individuals who might join the coalition. For nurses who tend to think only of other nurses and nursing groups, the challenge is to think beyond our profession. Local employers, for example, might be interested in a participating in a consortium to develop a wellness program for their employees. Encourage participation from all who might benefit or—conversely—all who might be disadvantaged if a proposed change such as restrictions on nursing practice occurs. Health care employers might be solicited for help to defeat legislation that would diminish their ability to assign and use nurses.

The third step is to determine the specific goal. The goal must be clearly and simply stated. All partners must be involved in this decision.

BOX 8-1

Steps for Building Coalitions

1. Identify the issue or problem.
2. Suggest potential groups or individuals for membership.
3. Determine the coalition's specific goal.
4. Decide on the coalition's time frame.

Anything left unstated could result in miscommunication or disagreement later. Sometimes, in the rush to gain support, important or controversial aspects are left out of the discussion to minimize discomfort and ensure agreement. Although detailed objectives needn't be stated at the outset, the goal itself should be clear and agreed upon by all members.

The time frame for the coalition's work follows. Then other potential partners or supporters are identified, along with detractors and those who might decline support. Finally, the group must decide the criterion that determines when the coalition is finished with its work: for example, the new program is begun, the grant is funded, or the political candidate is elected.

The group should disband when there is no longer a need for its collective action. Sometimes, members are reluctant to abandon the friendships and collegiality that may have developed among them, but unless the group has a purpose for remaining a coalition, it is best to free up the members to work with other groups. They could always reform in response to another issue or problem in the future.

To Go Formal or Informal

A coalition may be as informal as gathering a few colleagues at lunch and soliciting their interest in supporting or defeating a proposal before a committee due to meet that afternoon. Once the meeting is over and the decision has been made, this loose collection of individuals ceases to exist as a coalition.

On the other hand, a coalition can be as formal and long lasting as a standing committee or subcommittee, as described previously. It all depends on the goal or problem, the people or groups involved, and the situation. The most important point to remember is that a coalition can accomplish more than any one individual alone. That in itself is reason enough to participate in coalitions.

What You Know Now

You have learned that relationships are the building blocks of connections with others. You know that there are a number of ways that you can know others and become known by them. Small talk skills, attending professional meetings, and participating in social media and online discussion groups all help you build and use a network of contacts. You learned that building a network is a career-long strategy that can help you as well as others in your network. You know that you can compete with or support others and that neither should detract from the relationship. Finally, you learned that coalitions can do what you alone cannot do and that coalitions are invaluable in furthering nursing's goals.

You are ready to make connections and build coalitions!

Tools for Making Connections and Building Coalitions

1. Look for opportunities to use small talk at work and in personal environments. Assess how well you did.
2. Think about ways you can give to others. Follow up when the opportunity occurs.
3. Sign up on social media sites, explore blogs, and participate in online discussion groups.
4. Attend meetings of your professional association and other events.
5. Consider establishing a coalition to serve a purpose in your professional or personal life.
6. Review debts you owe and those owed to you. Remind yourself of those obligations when you need a favor or one is asked of you.

Learning Activities

1. Role-play small talk with a colleague or friend. Pretend you have just met. See how many of the skills described in this chapter you can use. You can use an observer to report, and each of you can report your experience as well. Think of ways you can improve your ability to use small talk.
2. Using Table 8-2, make a list of your professional and personal networks. Share your list with a friend or classmate. See if you can add to your list during the next week.
3. Review the scenario described in the section "When to Support." How would you handle the situation? Ask one or more colleagues or classmates how they would handle it. Compare your answers.

References

Arvin, D. (2009). *It's not who you know—it's who knows you!* New York: Wiley.

Baber, A., & Waymon, L. (2007). *Make your contacts count: Networking know-how for business and career success* (2nd ed.). New York: AMACOM.

Ondash, E. (2010). Networking to advance your nursing career. Retrieved November 15, 2010, from http://www.NurseConnect.com

Web Resources

Barrow, G. Making connections: Connecting creates influence. Retrieved April 15, 2011, from http://ezinearticles.com/?Making-Connections---Connecting-Creates-Influence&id=5132682

Bentley, C. Networking meetings: 8 rules for making connections. Retrieved April 15, 2011, from http://ezinearticles.com/?Networking-Meetings---8-Rules-For-Making-Connections&id=91927

Larson, J. The do's and don'ts of social media for nurses. Retrieved April 18, 2011, from http://www.nursezone.com/printArticle.aspx?articleID=36754

Thomas, E. 50 terrific social sites for nurses. Retrieved April 15, 2011, from http://www.nursingschools.net/blog/2009/07/50-terrific-social-sites-for-nurses/

CASE STUDY

Making Connections

Juan arrived at the community health nurses' conference and chose the sessions he planned to attend. "How to hold the most successful vaccination clinics" and "How to build relationships with your patients in the public health setting" were two of his selections.

That evening, Juan attended the opening night reception, mingled with other attendees, and visited vendor booths in the exhibit hall. At the poster presentations, he met Emily, a health department nurse. Her poster discussed ways to build a positive attitude and improve teamwork within the health department.

"I'd like to try some of your ideas in my public health clinic," Juan told Emily. "Could you tell me how you implemented some of these ideas in your setting? How did you, for example, create an expert list?"

"That was an especially successful strategy. In order to create the list of experts—team members and what they were best at—I had to poll each person. As team leader, that gave me a chance to interact one-on-one with my team in a positive way as they described their expertise."

"So then everyone knows the right person to ask if they have a specific question about some aspect of patient care," Juan said. "That's a great idea. Thanks. I'm going to try that at my department."

After talking for a while longer, Emily learned that Juan had done extensive work in setting up multiple vaccination clinics all over his city. "Our health department has been charged with something similar in our community," she said. "Can you give me some ideas of how we might set up flu clinics in our city?"

Juan was glad to help.

Emily asked Juan for his contact information so that they could continue to talk in the future. "I'd be happy to help you implement your team building strategies as well," she offered.

Juan was pleased to have made a new network contact at the conference. He was also surprised that he had skills and knowledge to offer Emily, just as she did for him. They set up a time to talk over the phone two weeks after the conference ended. After this call, Emily and Juan began to communicate regularly via e-mail. Juan realized how valuable a nursing network connection is to being successful.

9

Negotiating for What You Want

The goal of negotiation is to build bridges, not walls.

NICOLE SCHAPIRO

In this chapter, you will learn:

- What is involved in negotiation
- How to prepare for a negotiation
- How to conduct a negotiation meeting
- What to do following a negotiation meeting
- What can go wrong in a negotiation

WHAT IS NEGOTIATION?

The purpose of negotiation is to decide on a course of action agreeable to two or more parties when the parties have different goals. Negotiations occur daily. Buying a car, determining a salary, and complaining about a defective product all require negotiating skills. Some are spontaneous (e.g., "Will you cover my patients while I run an errand?"); others are more structured (e.g., employee grievance). Misconceptions about negotiation, however, are common.

Process versus Content

The process of negotiation is often confused with its content. The process is how the negotiation is structured. The content is the issue to be decided, the price to be determined, or the compensation to be paid. Both process and content are important for negotiations to be successful, but the process is sometimes ignored. How the negotiation is structured, however, sets the stage for the content.

Negotiation is one of the games played in the world of work, as described in Chapter 2. Negotiation has rules, and the rules determine how the game is played. The rules include who participates, when and where the negotiation takes place, how opposing views are presented and considered, and how a final decision is made. The rules may be implicit, which most negotiations are, or explicit, such as when spelled out in a collective bargaining agreement.

Negotiating Doesn't Equal Winning

Novice negotiators sometimes make the mistake of assuming that if they negotiate, they will win. Not so. Negotiation involves give and take, understanding what others want, and a willingness to find a solution that meets everyone's needs. Negotiation is not easy and not entered into lightly or without preparation.

For the Novice Nurse

You've been negotiating all your life. Negotiation in your professional life is no different than a teen offering to clean up his or her room in exchange for using the car. But the stakes are bigger. Your salary is one. It makes the difference in what you can afford to have and do. Some content in this chapter will be new to you. You have an opportunity to learn what an experienced nurse said "took years to learn."

Just think how far ahead you'll be!

Positional Bargaining versus Principled Negotiation

Bargaining from a position is the most common form of negotiation—and the one most likely to be unsuccessful. According to the groundbreaking work at the Harvard Negotiation Project, positional bargaining occurs when each side takes a position and argues for it and both make concessions to reach a compromise (Ury, 2008). Everyone has to give up and give in, and nobody wins. Furthermore, the relationship between the parties may be irreparably damaged, as anyone who has experienced an acrimonious settlement knows.

Principled negotiation focuses on the problem rather than the individuals or their positions, generates many possibilities before decisions are made, and bases results on an objective standard (Lyons, 2007). Principled negotiation should improve (or at least not damage) relationships, should be able to be settled in a timely fashion, and should meet the reasonable goals of all parties.

Group Characteristics and Their Effect on Negotiation

Ideally, negotiations should begin with all participants having comparatively equal status. In reality, however, that is seldom the case. In addition to differences in individuals' power, group differences may reflect perceived power inequalities and thus influence both the process and the outcome of the negotiation. These group characteristics include culture, race, gender, and age.

CULTURE. In some cultures, cooperation among members is more highly valued than individual achievement. When people from such a culture attempt to negotiate with individuals who have an orientation toward individual accomplishment, the two groups may have difficulty coming to agreement, due to their different perspectives.

RACE. Historical causes or stereotyping of certain groups may overtly or subtly influence how people of different races perceive each other and their inequitable power relationships, regardless of whether these differences exist.

GENDER. Similar to racial preconceptions, gender differences can influence negotiations. Women may feel like they have less power and attempt to offset their disadvantage by sabotaging the negotiating process, for example, and men may believe that they hold all the power and attempt to circumvent the negotiating process.

AGE. Generational differences also affect negotiations. Older, experienced nurses may be resistant to change (Malleo, 2010); younger nurses (Generation X) may welcome it. Generation Y (born after 1980) may be especially open to technological change (Swenson, 2008).

All these characteristics may interfere with the negotiating process. Recognizing that such variations exist may help participants understand their differences without letting them impede the negotiating process.

Negotiating Strategies

Legal nurse consultant Vickie Milazzo suggests strategies for negotiating (2010).

1. ***Ask for everything at the beginning.*** State your request up front. You can't change your mind halfway through the negotiation and ask for more.
2. ***Ask for more than you think you can get.*** This advice may sound as if it's the opposite of the previous recommendation, but it's not. It's an expansion of that strategy, and it's the hallmark of a good negotiator.

3. ***Don't be too fast to agree.*** Stop and think about the offer. It may be more than you expected—or less. Take time to decide whether it's acceptable.
4. ***Do not become emotional.*** Try to appear detached, even if that's difficult. The emotional participant loses points; the unemotional one gains them.
5. ***Don't assume that your bargaining power is weak because you want more than the other party.*** Uneven power positions can taint your perception. Don't let them.
6. ***Never say anything "off the record."*** What's said is said. There's no redo in negotiations.

THE NEGOTIATION

Throughout the course of your career, you will encounter numerous opportunities to negotiate with peers, supervisors, and subordinates. Some of these negotiations will be initiated by others and some by you. Regardless of the issue, the setting, or the initiator, negotiating successfully requires preparation, participation, and followup.

Preparing to Negotiate

The first step in a negotiation—preparation—is the one most likely to be ignored or to be sacrificed by busy people under the pressure of time. It is, however, the most important. The more information you have about the issue and the people involved, the better armed you are to offer workable suggestions and make wise decisions. Furthermore, you will be able to judge the give and take of participants throughout the negotiation. Preparation is key to a successful negotiation.

COLLECTING INFORMATION. Information can be gathered from a number of sources in addition to your own personal knowledge of the issue and the participants. Authoritative sources in nursing and health care can be used, including journals; books; local, state, and federal data; online reference; and experts (to name a few). Online library searches and databases, as well as the ability to contact experts online, make gathering information simpler and more available than a just a few years ago. Analyzing the data collected, however, requires skill, and the sheer mass of information makes the task challenging. Nonetheless, doing so prepares you to be able to begin the negotiation and to have additional information available as the negotiation proceeds. One caveat, however, must be offered. You will never have enough information, and if you waited until you did, the opportunity would be lost.

THE MEETING BEFORE THE MEETING. Remember the meeting before the meeting described in Chapter 5? This behind-the-scenes work is important in negotiations as well.

Once you have information assembled, categorized, and analyzed, it is time to meet with a few key individuals. Let's assume that you are going into a negotiation with several others from your unit or department. Two or more groups negotiating for a mutually beneficial arrangement is a likely scenario in most workplace negotiations.

Your group should get together, discuss their goals for the negotiation, and consider the information collected. Various suggestions that might come from the other parties should be considered. Ideas that might meet the opposing group's goals may emerge from this discussion. Role-playing the part of the opposition sometimes is useful to clarify issues and propose solutions.

Even in less-structured situations, chatting with a few key people may help identify issues or problems that they or others may have so that you can discuss these issues with them or contact others to do the same. Canvassing people you think might have opposing points of view can be valuable as well. They can raise issues you might not have considered, and you can use that information to craft your proposal.

Scheduling the Meeting

PARTICIPANTS. In most cases, each side of the negotiation decides upon the participants for their side. In general, individuals needed to approve or implement the decision participate in the meeting. Higher-level administrators needed for approval, however, would not attend unless their counterparts also attended. The university president might not be present at a negotiating meeting between the nursing school dean and his counterpart in another school, even though the president would be involved in any decisions about a joint program between the two schools.

Sometimes, such as in a union negotiation, the agreement spells out who will attend. In other situations, the two groups negotiate to decide attendees. Since it is seldom possible to get a group of busy people together at the same time, decisions must be made about whether substitute representatives are allowed (and if so, which representatives), and if the meeting must take place because of the time frame or other pressures, who can be left out.

MEETING LOCATION. Where the meeting is held is an important decision. Generally, the individual or group initiating the negotiation goes to the opposing side's location. You go to an auto dealer's showroom to buy a car; the dealer doesn't come to you. If you want to ask your boss for a raise, you go to your boss. The decision gets fuzzy, however, if there is some ambiguity about who wants what from whom or if the negotiation is expected to be acrimonious. In these instances, the meeting place may become a negotiation in itself.

A neutral location, if possible, is preferred in any circumstance, but that is seldom possible. If two hospitals are negotiating about exchanging services, it makes sense to meet at one or the other. In an unequal power situation, a group might decide to meet in a location favored by the person with less power, thereby equalizing the relative influence of opponents.

After the location is decided, the meeting room must be selected. Ideally, the room is easily found and large enough for everyone to sit around a table, the room temperature is comfortable for most participants, and it is close to restrooms. Nearby food service is also helpful.

LENGTH OF THE MEETING. One hour is an appropriate length of time for most meetings. If the meeting might run longer, it's a good idea to schedule a break after an hour. Participants can stretch their legs, use the facilities, refresh their drinks, and—most important—have time to consider the discussion. If negotiations become heated, a break may help dispel the tension.

MEETING DAY AND TIME. A number of decisions must be made regarding when to meet. Scheduling a meeting on Friday at 4:00 P.M., for example, may be a way for one side to attempt to intimidate the other or to press for a quick solution. Try to meet at a time when most participants will not be rushed, but it's a good idea not to allow more time than needed, such as when lunch time approaches.

Sharing information by mail ahead of time is useful if a large amount of data are used or if people need time to read and consider information. Be careful, though, that not so much material is distributed that decisions are made before the meeting.

DETERMINING THE AGENDA. Deciding what is to be included on the agenda (and what is left out) and the order in which topics are to be discussed is critical to a successful negotiation. The agenda also is a way to control the negotiation. It can facilitate or harm the outcome.

Start by brainstorming all possible topics, narrow those down to essential ones, and place topics in the order most likely to result in the preferred outcome. Although a printed agenda carries weight in any meeting, the discussion can and will deviate from the topics listed. Think of an agenda as the framework for discussion. As the discussion progresses and new information and ideas are presented, the agenda or its order can be modified. The agenda is useful to keep the discussion on track. Just don't adhere to it so rigidly that natural solutions are ignored.

The Meeting

SEATING ARRANGEMENTS. The first decision when arriving at the meeting place is where everyone should sit. Usually, you have a choice of seats; sometimes seating is assigned.

Positions influence the discussion and often the outcome. The head of the table is a power position. The facilitator, if there is one, should sit there, or the leader of the host group might assume that position. The person with the least power should avoid the head of the table and the seat directly opposite.

Think about the other individuals. With whom do you want to be able to make eye contact? Whose body language do you want to be able to see? The tendency is to sit as far as possible from someone you don't like or are afraid will be negative. Don't do that. Sitting next to that person makes agreement more likely and shows that you are confident as well as brave.

Avoid the tendency for your group to sit on one side and the opponents on the other. Such seating implies an adversarial position before the discussion even begins.

IN THE BEGINNING. Participants can help ease the tension inherent in any negotiation by engaging in small talk, as described in the previous chapter. Serving drinks or snacks gives participants something to do until everyone arrives and is settled. The goal should be to make everyone feel comfortable, which helps encourage cooperation and fosters creativity in generating ideas.

Once greetings and introductions are completed, the meeting begins. If there is a facilitator who is not involved with either party, he or she conducts the meeting. Without a facilitator, the initiator of the negotiation usually begins by presenting the initiating side's perception of the issue, and the responder follows. If both groups are prepared and are committed to principle-centered negotiation, a positive outcome can be anticipated.

DURING THE MEETING. Two items are important to a successful outcome. One is clarity about the issue. Sometimes the two groups have different ideas about what the issue is. Participants must be certain that everyone understands the issue before suggesting possible solutions.

Keeping on track is the other essential. Balancing each person's desire to speak and present an opinion with the need to keep the discussion focused is not easy. Experienced facilitators and leaders can help, as can group members. Having a written agenda in front of each person also helps. Keep in mind, though, that everyone should have an opportunity to share information and opinion. Leaving some out of the discussion in an effort to keep on track is equally as defeating.

PRESENTING YOURSELF. Adequate preparation is the first step to presenting yourself as a confident, competent negotiator. Try to sweep your mind clear of distractions and focus on the discussion. Note your body language. Is it congruent with your thoughts and statements? If not, do you have a reason to want to communicate a different message? Remember, other people can read your expression and body language as well as hear your words. Be sure to send the messages you intend.

Dressing to fit the occasion and to be most like the leaders is a general rule. Just don't deviate too far from your usual style. You want to fit in and be associated with the winners, but you don't want your appearance to distract you or other people. Sometimes, though, you want to stand out; then your dress might differ from others. Those in the visual and performing arts, for example, are expected to dress more flamboyantly than bankers, and academics are more casual than business people.

Female attorneys have been known to purposely appear delicate and feminine when they go into the most hard-nosed negotiations in order to throw off the opposition. Television interviewers may do the same. Regardless, you need to be comfortable enough that you can concentrate on the discussion and not on your appearance.

Attend to the discussion as it progresses, listen with an open mind to others' ideas, and encourage everyone to participate. Recall information from your preparation and use it as the necessity arises. Pay attention to how you are speaking—such as tone of voice—not just your words. You are building relationships with everyone there, and they will retain an impression of you long after this negotiation ends.

Take notes as needed, but don't pay so much attention to note taking that you can't participate. Usually, someone is assigned to record the discussion. You will be able to review the minutes at a later time. If, however, you are concerned that your opponents will try to control the content of the minutes or might intentionally forget some parts of the agreement, plan to jot down important points immediately after the meeting.

ENDING OR DELAYING. Successful negotiations come to an obvious conclusion. Participants agree on the next step, and everyone knows it's time to go. That doesn't always happen, of course. Sometimes it's best to delay a decision, gather more information, or allow participants to have time to consider the options. Delay doesn't mean that you abandon the project; it just means that more time is needed. Be willing to delay if it's appropriate, even if you had hoped for a final decision. Remember the quote at the beginning of the chapter: "The goal of negotiation is to build bridges, not walls."

At the closing, certain issues must be settled: what each person is assigned to do, in what time frame, and when and how everyone will be apprised. Whether there is to be a next step and if so, what that step should be is also determined.

FOLLOWUP. A meeting after the meeting (Chapter 6) gives you and your colleagues an opportunity to see where you stand vis-à-vis the decisions made and to regroup if the outcome was unsatisfactory. It also helps clarify any misunderstandings and confirm each person's assignment. Individually and together, members can evaluate their own participation in the meeting with the goal of improving their negotiating skills in the future. This is also the time to write down important points so that you can recall them later. To become a savvy negotiator, evaluate yourself every time you have a chance to participate in a negotiation.

Box 9-1 describes a successful negotiation.

BOX 9-1
Scenario of a Negotiation

A college of nursing decided to establish a nurse-managed clinic in order to offer clinical experiences for nurse practitioner students and practice for faculty. The administrator of a local hospital indicated an interest in cooperating with the college. She thought such an endeavor might help them avoid long waits in their emergency room for patients seeking nonemergency acute care.

A meeting was scheduled between the college's representatives and the hospital's. The business officer, the dean, and the faculty member designated to be the clinic's director from the college were scheduled to attend; the hospital administrator, the financial officer, the emergency room nursing supervisor, and the chief medical officer were slated to attend from the hospital. The meeting was a week away, and the dean assigned her business officer and the director of the proposed clinic the task of collecting information in preparation for the meeting.

Some of the information they collected included: how much time faculty would devote to practicing in the clinic, what arrangements other schools of nursing had made in similar circumstances, and the results of the other arrangements, especially monetary compensation. They polled their own faculty members for interest and determined how many hours each week students would be in the clinic. They found out that other schools had been successful with nurse-managed clinics under two conditions: that the school was compensated for care provided and that they were able to enhance faculty members' salaries with additional income.

On the other side, the hospital administrator asked her financial officer to find out how much the nonemergency care cost them over the past six months, the past year, and the past two years. She also talked with the chief medical officer to determine her willingness to provide backup medical supervision for the clinic, which would alleviate the excessive load in the ER. The ER physician agreed. The financial officer agreed that this would be a positive step for the hospital, providing that the monetary arrangements would benefit the hospital. The hospital representatives learned that most of the nonemergency care they were providing in the ER was not reimbursed; if they could pay less to the college for that care than they spent on salaries, such an arrangement would be financially sound.

The meeting was held at 2:00 P.M. in the hospital administrator's conference room. Introductions were made as people arrived. Everyone took seats around the oval-shaped table after getting soft drinks or coffee.

The agenda was as follows:

1. Rationale for nurse-managed clinic (dean)
2. Advantages to the hospital (administrator)
3. Advantages to the community
4. Suggestions for staffing, equipment, and funding
5. Potential problems
6. Discussion of possible solutions
7. Dean and administrator agree on final decision, if possible
8. Follow-up assignments

The meeting went as planned, but unforeseen problems emerged. Space near the ER was limited, so considerable discussion ensued among the hospital representatives about various uses of space around the hospital. As the discussion veered away from the agenda, the administrator brought the discussion back to the topic at hand and a nearby site was identified.

The medical officer balked at calling the clinic "nurse-managed," but eventually she realized the name was appropriate because it would be staffed by nurses and a recent survey had shown that the public rated nurses high on trust. The public relations advantage was apparent.

How to cover the clinic during school vacations was another issue that everyone had failed to identify. Instead of a problem, though, it appeared to help settle the issue of how to increase faculty compensation by paying faculty to cover the clinic during the college's scheduled vacations.

Various other issues were discussed and reasonable solutions proposed. The dean and administrator agreed to meet with their respective legal counsels to consider the details of the agreement, but all left the meeting convinced that a nurse-managed clinic would be established at the hospital.

Negotiating from a Distance

For today's busy people, conferencing at a distance is easier than ever. Virtual meetings may be held via phone conference calls, online, or as a video conference, which offers the advantage of being able to see expressions, gestures, and other indicators of body language.

Audio conferencing from phone and computer services such as http://www.GoToMeeting.com allows participants to simultaneously view the same computer screen, share presentations, and edit documents while speaking by phone or via their computer's microphone and speakers. In addition, the call can be recorded and the recording downloaded as needed.

Similar to in-person meetings, decisions must be made concerning the participants, when the meeting will be held, who will lead it, and what will be on the agenda. Usually, these issues are decided early by the leaders of each group.

Participants connect online, enter the video conference room, or join the phone call in the same way they would enter a meeting room, usually one or a few at a time. Making small talk is usually held to a minimum but enough time should be allowed to welcome everyone and to answer any immediate questions participants have.

On a phone conference, the leader must pay close attention to a lack of response. Protracted silence may convey reflection, distraction, or disapproval. Participants may be interrupted or may be trying to do other work, such as read text messages or answer e-mail. Asking people directly for questions or comments can help refocus participants' attention. A specific agenda and a commitment to keeping the meeting moving helps to keep participants from mentally detaching, whether on the phone, online, or by video.

WHAT CAN GO WRONG

As in any human endeavor, many things can go wrong, even with the best intentions of all involved. Following are a few of the reasons negotiations are unsuccessful (Donaldson, 2007):

1. ***Negotiation starts too soon.*** Members might not be prepared. Materials haven't been obtained or information analyzed. Partners have not been canvassed. Participants must feel comfortable that they are ready to negotiate, but others may be pressing for a quick response. Be honest. Admit you aren't ready and use the occasion to inquire about the opposition's position.
2. ***The wrong people are involved.*** The person at the meeting may not be the appropriate representative to participate in the negotiation or may be unable to answer questions or make a commitment. Always make certain that you are negotiating with the appropriate representative.
3. ***Lack of commitment or involvement.*** Participants may deter success if they are unwilling to share information, maintain a rigid position even in the face of competing information, or harbor a hidden agenda. A hidden agenda disguises an ulterior motive. One participant might be trying to show off in front of his superiors, for example; another might be trying to find out your strategy so that she can use it herself. Keep your antenna out for hints that all is not as it seems.
4. ***The group digresses.*** The tendency to digress and get off the topic is powerful in any group discussion. The complexity of most negotiations makes this even more a possibility. The agenda and your own preparation and notes can help the group return to the topic at hand.
5. ***Emotional outbursts.*** Many negotiations deal with sensitive issues about which participants feel strongly. Negotiations also show people at their most vulnerable, often in front of colleagues. When things don't go well, anger or tears may result. If that happens, a decision must be made about continuing or delaying the meeting. Sometimes taking a short break helps to relieve the tension and gets people back on track.
6. ***Failing to close.*** A close cousin to closing too soon is failing to close in a timely fashion. Continuing beyond the closing point may lead to dissembling the agreement, requiring participants to begin again. Also, assignments and follow-up dates must be set. Without a clear understanding of everything to be done and a schedule, a successful decision would fail to be implemented.

What can you do if you lose? Sometimes, in spite of our best preparation, our position fails to be persuasive. Losing is not easy, but you can turn it into an advantage. If the discussion seems to be going against your interests, think about what you might want in the future and if the participants are in a position to help you.

Remember quid pro quo discussed in Chapter 2? You are now in a position to give in, at the same time reminding others that they owe you. If you think you're about to lose, you can use your acquiescence as a bargaining tool, saying that you'll let them have this if you can have something else you need now. Savvy players know that you've racked up some chips, that if they don't have something for you now you'll come calling in the future, and that they'll be obligated to honor their debt. Remember that.

What You Know Now

You have learned that negotiation is complex and involves both the process (how the negotiation is structured) and the content (the issue to be decided). You know that just because you negotiate doesn't mean you'll win. You also know that negotiations should be based on principles of fairness and consideration and that bargaining from a set position is unsatisfactory for everyone. You learned that adequate preparation is essential and that scheduling, location, meeting room, and seating arrangements can hinder or facilitate a successful negotiation. Structuring the agenda to adequately consider many alternatives and to settle on the best one is necessary for a positive outcome to be generated. Successful negotiations can be conducted from a distance. Finally, you learned about some situations that can interfere with successful negotiations.

You're ready to negotiate!

Tools for Negotiating

1. Be sure that you are prepared with necessary information before going into any negotiation.
2. Be mentally and physically ready to negotiate.
3. Be sensitive to a hidden agenda, and take steps to offset its influence on the group.
4. Evaluate your participation after every negotiating session. Think about what you could have done differently.

Learning Activities

1. To evaluate your negotiating skills, rate yourself on the following:
   I understand that negotiation means compromise.
   I prepare for negotiations with information and a positive attitude.
   I maintain respect for all parties during negotiation.
   I am a good listener.
   I can look at an issue from another's perspective.
   I remain open to suggestions.
   I am a good problem solver.
   I attack problems, not people.
   I can distinguish facts from opinions.
   I understand that negotiations are not always successful.
   I am confident in my own abilities.
   I am a team player.

I keep in mind that relationships may remain after negotiations end.
I use silence appropriately.
I get clear agreement before leaving.
I follow up as agreed.

2. Recall a negotiation involving several people that went wrong. Were any of the reasons listed in the chapter why it was unsuccessful? What could you or others have done differently?
3. Recall your own experience with an unsuccessful negotiation involving one other person. What could you have done differently? Be specific. Role-play this negotiation with a colleague, using the principles presented in this chapter. Then role-play the same scenario, but this time play the role of your opponent. Share what you learned from both role-playing scenarios with classmates.

References

Donaldson, M. C. (2007). *Negotiating for dummies.* (2nd ed.). Hoboken, NJ: Wiley.

Lyons, C. (2007). *I win, you win: The essential guide to principled negotiation.* London: A&C Black.

Malleo, C. (2010). Each generation brings strengths, knowledge to nursing field: A nurse's journal. Retrieved November 19, 2010, from http://www.cleveland.com/healthfit/index.ssf/2010/02/each_generation_brings_strengt.html

Milazzo, V. (2010). 5 negotiation strategies for certified legal nurse consultants. Retrieved November 19, 2010, from http://www.legalnurse.com/vickiesblog/2010/01/5-negotiation-strategies-for-certified-legal-nurse-consultants/

Swenson, C. (2008). Next generation workforce. *Nursing Economics, 26*(1), 64–65.

Ury, W. (2008). *The power of a positive no.* New York: Bantam.

Web Resources

Dawson, R. Basic principles make you a smarter negotiator. Retrieved April 14, 2011, from http://ezinearticles.com/?Basic-Principles-Make-You-A-Smarter-Negotiator&id=104901

Mazmi, M. Effective method of negotiation. Retrieved April 14, 2011, from http://ezinearticles.com/?Effective-Method-of-Negotiation&id=1671981

Williams, G. Use the right negotiation style to be a winning negotiator. Retrieved April 11, 2011, from http://ezinearticles.com/?Use-the-Right-Negotiation-Style-to-Be-a-Winning-Negotiator&id=1252382

Williams, G. Negotiating right may not mean right now. Retrieved April 14, 2011, from http://ezinearticles.com/?Negotiating-Right-May-Not-Mean-Right-Now&id=1459661

CASE STUDY

Using Negotiating Skills

Pat, Margaret, and Hyereon worked together on the psychiatric care unit at Union Hospital. Their unit offered self scheduling, so each member of the team was allowed to request the days they would like to work each month.

The system worked well, and the staff enjoyed the autonomy they were allowed in choosing their schedule.

All staff members had to agree to work two Mondays and two Fridays each month and every third weekend, both Saturday and Sunday. Mondays and Fridays were the two hardest days to cover and were the busiest days on the unit. Staff members complained, saying that they would like to be able to break these days apart if they chose to and work them on different weekends. Pat, Margaret, and Hyereon agreed to work together on submitting this suggestion to management.

Before requesting a meeting time with the scheduling committee and the nurse manager, the three RNs assembled all information they thought would be necessary to convince them to try a schedule change. They composed mock schedules for when staff worked their weekend days consecutively and when they worked the same number of days but not consecutively.

They reminded their peers that all patient care shifts would still have to be covered. That might require someone to switch the weekend day if not enough staff are scheduled on another weekend day. The nursing team agreed that they could honor this commitment.

Pat, Margaret, and Hyereon practiced what they would present to the decision makers. The three nurses scheduled a time to meet with the scheduling committee and the nurse manager on a day and time that was conducive to the schedule of these individuals.

They shared their proposal with the group and presented the mock schedules showing shift coverage currently and in the proposed system. They assured the committee and the manager that other staff agreed to be flexible to meet the unit's staffing needs if this new scheduling method was tried. They reported that this new system was highly desired by the nursing staff and that they believed it would increase job satisfaction for the staff.

"I appreciate the time and effort you three have put into preparing this proposal," said Hadley, the nurse manager. Several members of the scheduling committee nodded.

"We'll discuss this and get back to you," Hadley said.

A few weeks later, Hadley reported back. "We don't know if this will work, but we're willing to try it as a pilot for the next three months and then evaluate how well it worked. Will you agree that we'll return to the current system if it doesn't work?"

The nurses looked at each other. Pat spoke for them. "Yes. If it doesn't work to your satisfaction, then we'll go back to consecutive weekend shifts."

"If it works as well as you three think it will," Hadley said, "then we could continue using it for weekend scheduling."

Pat, Margaret, and Hyereon agreed: their negotiation was a success.

10

Dealing with Difficult People and Situations

The most important single ingredient in the formula of success is the knack of getting along with people.

THEODORE ROOSEVELT

In this chapter, you will learn:

- How to identify difficult situations and individuals
- How to evaluate the seriousness of a situation
- How to confront problem situations
- How to handle bullying
- What to do if the situation turns dangerous

DEALING WITH PROBLEMS

On your way to becoming influential, you will inevitably be faced with problems involving troublesome people and challenging situations. Some of these situations are more difficult than others, but learning how to confront difficult people and situations is an important skill that can help you safely traverse the minefields of life and work.

We all have known difficult people and have been confronted by troublesome situations. You can probably easily think of a few examples. Unfortunately, these situations often take us by surprise, and only in retrospect do we realize how we could have handled the event better.

By not initiating difficult conversations, patients can be endangered, according to a study by Vitalsmarts (2005). The researchers found seven areas where health care workers found it difficult to speak up, including seeing colleagues make mistakes, perform incompetently, disrespect others, break rules, fail to support colleagues, exhibit poor teamwork, and micromanage inappropriately. So it is essential that you learn to handle challenging situations—no matter how uncomfortable they make you.

This chapter covers a variety of behavior and situations that you may encounter, but we will by no means cover the multitude of problems you will face over the course of a career. The goals here are to provide some clues to identifying difficult situations and personalities early and to offer strategies to handle most of them.

Difficult People

We might be working side by side with difficult people or sometimes they seem to appear out of nowhere, undercutting our work and our life. They may be our bosses, our colleagues, or our subordinates. We may often be in conflict with physicians and other health care professionals when our ideas and theirs are at odds. Patients and their families can prove difficult, as can students and instructors. Members of the public also may be combative and difficult. There is no end to the people we might face who behave in ways we wish they wouldn't and who can bring immense trouble and grief into our lives. Fortunately, they are usually the exception, not the rule.

Difficult Situations

Difficult situations can vary from minor verbal altercations to dangerous attacks. Verbal abuse, online or text bullying, physical threats, and sexual harassment are very real in today's workplace, including universities and health care facilities. Being attacked, ignored, or lied to is not uncommon. Some people become inadvertent victims of dirty tricks (see Chapter 6) or are faced with a person out of control. At some time, you may be confronted with legal problems, such as observing a licensure violation or a potential malpractice situation.

Ethical dilemmas abound in health care and are more common as increasingly better techniques to keep patients alive are developed. You may have a conflict with another individual, or you may be involved in conflicts among several others or groups. At times, you may be responsible for calming combatants or disciplining employees.

Some people are always difficult, and sometimes even the calmest of individuals become difficult in troubling situations. Any manner of human behavior you can imagine can happen. Learning strategies and tactics for ameliorating conflicts will help you face these situations with some measure of confidence.

For the Novice Nurse

Everyone faces difficult people and situations, and few of us knew how to deal with bullies and others. You are no different. All of us are reluctant to confront bullies and other difficult people and situations, even when the circumstances require it. Unlike new nurses who don't have this book, you can learn how to handle all of them.

Bullying

Bullying in the workplace isn't unique to nursing, but in a health care setting, bullying behaviors not only threaten the victim (called a "target") but pose a danger to patients as well (Stokowski, 2010). Called incivility, verbal abuse, or vertical or horizontal violence, all such behaviors are examples of bullying (Broome, 2008). Nurses report verbal abuse as the most frequent form of bullying (Christmas, 2007); senior nurses, managers, and physicians are the most likely perpetrators (Vessey, DeMarco, Gaffney, & Budin, 2009).

Bullying behaviors can range from mildly irritating to dangerously violent (Stokowski, 2010). Examples include:

Being ignored or given the "silent treatment"

Treated in a condescending or patronizing manner

Derogatory remarks within hearing

Dismissive body language, such as eye rolling

Ridicule, sarcasm

Verbal abuse

Sexual harassment

Physical attack

Bullies may be soft-spoken and may appear to be polite. They may even smile as they deliver their zingers. They rely on their power, actual or perceived, to make you do what they want by intimidating you.

"Intervene quickly to prevent minor conflicts from escalating," recommends Dellasega (2009). Broome (2008) advises both victims and those who witness abuse to confront the abuser, whom she calls "sharks" and "bullies"; see Table 10-1. Often witnesses fear becoming targets themselves. Work isn't for the wimpy, regardless of how difficult it is to stand up for a coworker.

Organizational efforts to reduce workplace bullying have been launched (Trossman, 2010). The Joint Commission recommends zero tolerance of disruptive or abusive behavior (Joint Commission, 2008). In addition, the American Nurses Association 2010 House of Delegates passed a resolution to combat hostility, abuse, and bullying in the workplace (2010).

Healthy workplace bills that would allow workers to sue for harm from abusive treatment are being considered in several states (Stokowski, 2010).

TABLE 10-1 Rules for Dealing with Sharks and Bullies

1. Assume that all fish are sharks.
2. Do not bleed.
3. Control your anger.
4. Counter aggression promptly.
5. Avoid ingratiating behaviors.
6. Use anticipatory retaliation.
7. Document attacks.

Adapted from Broome, B. A. (2008). Dealing with sharks and bullies in the workplace. *ABNF Journal*, Winter, 28–30. Used with permission.

As widespread reports of abuse surface, it is hoped that swift legal action will offer redress for victims. In the meantime, keep alert for instances of bullying, prepare yourself to counter any attack, and document whatever occurs (Lazoritz & Carlson, 2008).

STRATEGIES FOR MANAGING DIFFICULT SITUATIONS

Evaluate the Situation

There are numerous potentially difficult situations. People who are hostile, arrogant, deceptive, manipulative, rude, self-seeking, rigid, procrastinate, uncommunicative, or critical populate every workplace, and, at some time or another, you will encounter such people. Sometimes you will be driven to distraction by their behavior; other times you will be able to get around them or ignore them. To decide whether to respond, ask yourself the following questions:

- What will likely happen if I intervene in the situation?
- How might my response affect the other person?
- How might my intervention affect others in our workgroup or my institution?
- What might happen if I don't intervene?

(If you think the situation might become dangerous, see the section "If the Confrontation Turns Dangerous" later in this chapter.)

Decide to Intervene

What do you want to accomplish? The outcome you want determines your decision to intervene and how you intervene. If one of your subordinates is behaving in an objectionable, hostile or harassing manner, you need to intervene. If you don't, other employees will resent the lack of intervention and might begin to emulate the negative behavior. Whenever someone's behavior interferes with the functioning of your area of responsibility, you must intervene.

Sometimes problems involve two or more people. If, for example, two employees are feuding, their arguments might spill over and involve others who may side with one or the other. These situations must be defused before mistakes are made or high-performing people leave. If you are unable to solve a problem, contact the person immediately superior to you in the management chain, such as your immediate supervisor, for assistance.

If your problem involves your supervisor (or your instructor, if you are a student), you need to speak directly to the person first. Give him or her a chance to explain the situation. You may be able to see the issue from a broader perspective after this discussion. If you aren't satisfied after speaking with the person directly involved, consider going to the next level, such as the institution's chief nurse or the school's dean. If you are still not satisfied, you can file a formal grievance.

Universities have grievance procedures, and workplaces with collective bargaining agreements have specified steps to lodge grievances. If you are not satisfied with the outcome of the grievance and you strongly believe your position is correct, you can consider going outside the organizational structure and initiating legal proceedings. Be sure you want to do that, though. A legal proceeding is an expensive endeavor that requires emotional fortitude and may not be successful. You, of course, can consider leaving the institution or changing colleges.

Once you have decided to intervene, it is best to do so as soon as possible before the problem escalates. Then you must decide where to deal with the situation. Privacy is of utmost importance. No one wants to be embarrassed in front of other people; embarrassing someone is likely to be ineffective, as well. So what can you do? It's time to learn how to confront a problem situation.

CONFRONTATION

Confronting another person is probably everyone's least favorite task. Many of us try to put it off, hoping the problem will go away on its own, or try to get someone else to handle the problem. Wishing problems away doesn't work; they often come back to haunt us and may escalate when left unresolved.

(Before reading any farther, take the self-assessment pretest in Box 10-1.)

Four Steps to Confronting Others

Regardless of how many times you have confronted people, each occurrence produces anxiety. Good preparation can help. Table 10-2 lists the steps of confrontation.

First, determine the problem. What exactly is bothering you about the person's behavior? Are you tired of waiting for the colleague who is perpetually late for work? Do you have to discipline an employee? Do you think your instructor has been unfair? Using these examples, here are some ways to begin the confrontation:

BOX 10-1

Pretest Your Confrontation Skills

1. I often get my feelings hurt by other people.
2. I overlook other people's behavior if I don't like it.
3. It helps me to tell someone about another's behavior rather than talking with the person directly.
4. I often apologize for things that aren't my fault.
5. If something goes wrong, it's seldom my fault.
6. I try to control myself when I'm angry, but often I can't help yelling.
7. I expect other people to recognize when I'm upset.
8. If I tell someone I'm upset, I'm afraid the person will not like me anymore.
9. If I have to tell people I'm upset, I imply that the problem is my fault so they won't get their feelings hurt.

Describe the problem

"When you're late, change of shift report is delayed."

"We have had several meetings about your behavior, but it hasn't changed."

"My test scores were high, yet I didn't get an A."

Explain how that behavior is affecting you

"Patient care is delayed in the morning."

"Other staff members and patients have complained about your behavior."

"I don't think that my grade is fair."

Say what you want to have change

"I want you to be at work on time."

"I want your behavior to change."

"I want my grade to accurately reflect my work."

TABLE 10-2 Steps in Confrontation
1. Identify the problem.
2. Tell how that problem is affecting you.
3. Say what you want to have happen.
4. Ask if the other person is willing to do what you asked.
5. Decide on follow-up.

Ask if the other person is willing to do what you asked

"Will you try to be at work on time from now on?"

"Will you try to change your behavior?"

"Will you review my work and see how I may improve that grade?"

It is unusual that this last step works as simply as described. More often, this step is a negotiating position, such as, "I don't know if I can make on time every day. Maybe I could start a half hour later and stay a half hour later." Then you might explain why that would not work, and depending on the person's response, you might need to take the next step, such as writing the person up (if he or she is a subordinate) or going to your supervisor.

Finally, decide on follow-up

If you are disciplining an employee who agrees to change his or her behavior, set a time to check back again to see whether the behavior has indeed changed. If your instructor agrees to review your work to determine whether your grade is correct, find out when he or she will have a decision for you. Then follow up in a timely manner. Nothing can undo a positive change faster than thinking that the improvement went unnoticed, especially if only negative behavior is noticed.

One situation that often tempts people to intervene is when a problem develops that does not directly involve you but is annoying nonetheless. Take, for example, the coworker who is habitually late. Your responsibility ends when you explain how the tardiness affects you and ask for the behavior to change. Disciplining the employee is his or her supervisor's job. There is nothing wrong with trying to change the behavior by confronting the person or with reporting the problem. Just recognize that your influence alone may not change the behavior.

Problems in Confronting Others

WEAKENING YOUR MESSAGE. Remember the discussion in Chapter 5 about women's tendencies to weaken their statements with qualifiers? Starting a statement with "I don't know if you thought of this, but . . . " or ending a statement with "although I'm sure you've thought of it" lower the impact of your ideas. Certain words do the same. "Kind of," "sort of," "really," "truly," and "very" are examples of qualifiers, along with excessive use of noncommittal sounds, such as "um" or "uh huh." "I'm sorry, but . . . " should not be used unless you intend to apologize, not to soften your words.

You can weaken your message if you show nervousness. Nervousness can undermine your effectiveness as surely as using qualifiers before or after your message. Good preparation helps to reduce the jitters. Experience with successful (though no less painful) confrontations does also. It gives you some confidence that you can confront someone in a positive way. Try memorizing your first few words and concentrate on those as you begin. You will find that once you start to speak, your nervousness will diminish.

TABLE 10-3 Hierarchy of Directness

I want. I have to have. (Most direct)
I would like. I would prefer. (Less direct)
Could you? Is it possible? (Least direct)

Pachter, B., & Magee, S. (2001). *The power of positive confrontation: The skills you need to know to handle conflicts at work, at home, and in life.* Cambridge, MA: Da Capo Press. Used with permission.

BEING TOO DIRECT. When you dive directly into the problem, you might catch the person so off guard that the immediate response is an angry retort. If the issue is charged with emotion and you want to ease into the discussion, preface your discussion of the problem with softening words or a smile (Zofi & Meltzer, 2007):

"You may not be aware of this, but . . . "

"I wanted to let you know something that's been bothering me."

On the other hand, if you soften it too much, the person may not take you seriously or may be able to turn the issue around so that it seems as if you did something wrong. A general rule is that you can be more direct with subordinates, including students; less direct with colleagues; and the least direct with your supervisor, including instructors. Examples are shown in Table 10-3.

DEALING WITH EMOTION. We all wish we could remain calm despite others' behavior, but as human beings, that's impossible. Police officers often face hostile or dangerous situations. They are trained to avoid any response that might irritate or encourage their attacker, whether someone is verbally abusing them or physically attacking them. You can learn some of the same skills with preparation and vigilance.

Sometimes we can remain calm but the other person erupts with emotion, either in anger or by crying. Both can make you feel as if you did something wrong, but you are not responsible for other people's emotions. Depending on the situation, you may need to get away (if you think you might be in danger), but more often you can help by remaining calm yourself.

Most people have a tendency to react to anger with anger, increasing the tension and escalating the problem. Don't try to explain or justify your position or deflect the rage against you. Let the storm pass. Make notes after the event, verify statements the person made to you, and—if possible—go back with a potential solution. Stick to solving the problem.

What should you do if you are overwhelmed with emotion? It is best to excuse yourself and come back when you are calmer. It helps to tell someone how you feel; that's perfectly acceptable in the workplace: "When you criticize me in front of patients, I feel embarrassed." You don't need to go into details; just state how a behavior affects you.

WANTING THE IMPOSSIBLE. Be sure that what you want is possible. If you ask your supervisor whether you can attend a conference during a week in which one person is on vacation and another is due to have surgery, it is doubtful that you will be able to attend without seriously compromising coverage on the unit. You might be able to suggest alternatives, such as agency help, but be prepared for your request to be denied. Ask yourself two questions: is he or she the right person to ask? Can the person do what I want?

Achieving balance in confronting others requires considerable thought ahead of time, including how you expect the person to respond and ways in which you might deal with these responses. Practice various scenarios until you feel comfortable. Realize that everyone dreads confrontations, including the person you plan to confront. (See Table 10-4 for some do's and don'ts of confrontation.)

When You Are Confronted

Many of the same rules apply when someone confronts you. The difference is that it is unexpected and you are unprepared. Learning the steps (see Table 10-2), though, can help you prepare to respond in these difficult situations.

First, evaluate the danger, which is more likely when you are being confronted by an angry or distraught person. Patients, their families, hospital visitors, and other staff are among the many potential attackers. Never try to handle a potentially dangerous situation by yourself. (See the following section, "If the Confrontation Turns Dangerous.")

If you are confronted with a situation that is not likely to become dangerous, the next step is to determine the problem. When people are upset, they often blurt out their frustration without identifying the problem. Wait, take a breath, and—when he or she stops talking—calmly ask them to describe the problem. Listen carefully while trying to discern the exact nature of the problem. It's likely that he or she will take the next step—telling you how the problem is affecting them—without prompting.

Decide whether this is a problem that you can and wish to handle. Someone else may be better able to fix the problem, or you may decide that this is not a situation in which you should become involved. In these cases,

TABLE 10-4 Do's and Don'ts in Confrontation

- DO define the problem.
- DON'T use "always" or "never."
- DO tell how the behavior affects you.
- DON'T get into other people's problems.
- DO say what you want to change.
- DON'T ask for the impossible.
- DO ask if the other person understands and agrees.

tell the person your decision, suggest someone else for them to contact, and wish them well. Often, just listening to the person's problem helps alleviate a stressful situation (which can be common in nursing). Remember what you learned about delivering the message to the right person in Chapter 2? It does little good to complain to a colleague about a situation that the colleague cannot fix; go to the person who can fix it.

If you are able to help, ask what the person wants to have happen. Sometimes a modest change will satisfy; other times, a major change is required. In the latter case, more people are probably necessary, and solving the problem will undoubtedly take some time.

If you decide that it is worth investing your time and political capital, you can get the process started. Involve the person with the solution as much as possible. For example, if you are confronted by a coworker and the two of you realize that your supervisor needs to be involved, send your coworker to set up the appointment. The problem is the coworker's, remember, and doing something to solve the problem invests him or her in the outcome. Ask your coworker if this is a satisfactory first step and agree on the next steps and a time frame for follow-up.

Here are some general guidelines for dealing with difficult people and situations:

- Focus on the problem, not the person.
- Keep control of your emotions or excuse yourself until you have control.
- If a hostile situation develops, consider postponing the meeting or discussion until a later time.
- Deal with the issue personally if written or verbal messages might be misconstrued.
- Keep conversations private, including only those directly involved.
- Record notes after an altercation that might develop into a legal problem. Reviewing your notes also gives you an opportunity to learn from the situation.
- Always be gracious, regardless of anyone else's behavior. Their behavior is theirs alone, as is the embarrassment.
- Remember that it's not personal; it's business. Drop it at the door when you leave work.

If the Confrontation Turns Dangerous

If you are physically in danger or if the situation might escalate and put you in harm's way, you must take immediate action. One way to evaluate the danger is watching body language. Law enforcement personnel use this assessment tool all the time. Positions to watch for are:

- Clenched fists
- Blank stare
- Fighting stance (one foot back with arm pulled back ready to strike)
- Arms raised in a fighting position

- Standing too close or advancing toward you
- Holding anything that might be used as a weapon, such as a pen, letter opener, heavy object, and, of course, any actual weapon, such as a knife or gun
- Overt intent (say that they intend to "kick your [body part]" or similar statements)
- Movement toward the exit to prevent you from leaving

Also, anyone under the influence of drugs or alcohol is unpredictable and potentially dangerous. If you notice any of these behaviors, get away as quickly as you can and report the incident to authorities. If someone at your institution does not take action, call the police. An actual or threatened assault is illegal. Never ignore it.

What You Know Now

You have learned about the array of difficult people and situations that you may encounter throughout the course of your career. You know how to evaluate situations for how serious these situations are and whether they require you to intervene. You can recognize bullying behaviors and know to intervene to prevent escalation. You have considered the steps for confronting others and when they confront you. You know how to determine whether a situation is dangerous and what to do if you encounter a threatening situation. You know that handling difficult people and situations takes preparation, practice, and experience.

Now that you've read the chapter, take the self-assessment posttest in Box 10-2.

BOX 10-2

Posttest Your Confrontation Skills

1. I look people in the eye when speaking to them.
2. My facial expression is consistent with what I am saying.
3. I do not point my finger at others when I speak.
4. I speak loudly enough for others to hear.
5. I do not giggle at the end of my sentences.
6. When talking with others, I do not play with my hair, tie, mustache, or jewelry; crack my knuckles; or play with my phone.
7. I don't slouch, sway, or lean when standing.
8. I know the proper distance to stand when speaking with others.
9. I'm aware of what gestures I'm using.
10. I show that I am listening to others.

Pachter, B., & Magee, S. (2001). *The power of positive confrontation: The skills you need to know to handle conflicts at work, at home, and in life.* Cambridge, MA: Da Capo Press. Used with permission.

Tools for Dealing with Difficult People and Situations

1. Learn to identify situations that require your intervention.
2. Deal with problems as soon as possible.
3. Learn confrontation skills and practice them.
4. Evaluate each confrontation for ways you could improve in the future.
5. Get away if a situation threatens to become or turns dangerous.

Learning Activities

1. Recall a confrontation you handled. Using the steps described in the chapter, evaluate how well you did. Can you think of any way you could have done it better? Jot down those strategies somewhere where you can refer to them now and then. The next time you have a confrontation to conduct, refer to your notes.
2. Recall a situation in which you were confronted. What happened? How did you handle it? Could you have done anything differently? Share your experience with a colleague or friend.
3. Role-play one of the situations in the previous activities with a partner. Then reverse and role-play a situation that your partner encountered. Share what you have learned from each other's experiences.

References

American Nurses Association. (2010). Hostility, abuse and bullying in the workplace. House of Delegates Resolution. *The Kansas Nurse, 85*(6), 17.

Broome, B. A. (2008, Winter). Dealing with sharks and bullies in the workplace. *ABNF Journal*, 28–30.

Christmas, K. (2007). Workplace abuse: Finding solutions. *Nursing Economics, 25*(6), 365–367.

Dellasega, C. A. (2009). Bullying among nurses. *American Journal of Nursing, 109* (1), 52–58.

Joint Commission. (2008, July 9). Behaviors that undermine a culture of safety. Retrieved October 15, 2010, from http://www.jointcommission.org/sentinel_event_alert_issue_40_behaviors_that_undermine_a_culture_of_safety/

Lazoritz, S., & Carlson, P. J. (2008). Don't tolerate disruptive physician behavior. *American Nurse Today, 3*(3). Retrieved November 22, 2010, from http://www.americannursetoday.com/Popups/ARticlePrint.aspx?id=7194

Pachter, B., & Magee, S. (2001). *The power of positive confrontation: The skills you need to know to handle conflicts at work, at home, and in life*. Cambridge, MA: Da Capo Press.

Stokowski, L. A. (2010). A matter of respect and dignity: Bullying in the nursing profession. Retrieved October 15, 2010, from http://www.medscape.com/viewarticle/729474

Trossman, S. (2010). Not "part of the job": Nurses seek an end to workplace violence. *The American Nurse* (November/December). Retrieved August 16, 2011 from http://www.nursingworld.org

Vessey, J. A., DeMarco, R. F., Gaffney, D. A., & Budin, W. C. (2009). Bullying of staff registered nurses in the workplace: A preliminary study for developing personal and organizational strategies for the transformation of hostile to healthy workplace environments. *Journal of Professional Nursing, 25*(5), 299–306.

VitalSmarts (2005). Silence kills: The seven crucial conversations in healthcare. Retrieved April 12, 2011, from http://www.silencekills.com/UPDL/SilenceKillsExecSummary.pdf

Zofi, Y. S., & Meltzer, S. (2007). Dealing with difficult people. *Nursing Homes/Long Term Care Management, 56*(8), 48–49.

Web Resources

Allen, B. R. 4 reasons to be timely with your confrontation. Retrieved April 22, 2011, from http://ezinearticles.com/?4-Reasons-to-Be-Timely-With-Your-Confrontation&id=3538789

Bartkus, J. Confrontation at work. Retrieved April 11, 2011, from http://ezinearticles.com/?Confrontations-at-Work&id=2599721

Borgatti, J. C. How to stay safe in a sometimes-scary world. *American Nurse Today, 4*(9). Retrieved April 11, 2011, from http://www.americannursetoday.com/Article.aspx?id=6036&fid=6002

Buppert, C. What should I do when bullied by someone higher up? Retrieved April 11, 2011, from http://www.medscape.com/viewarticle/735217

Maybin, S. To confront or not confront: What to say when you'd rather not say anything at all. Retrieved April 18, 2011, from http://ezinearticles.com/?To-Confront-or-Not-to-Confront?:--What-to-Say-When-Youd-Rather-Not-Say-Anything-At-All&id=465187

Rosenblatt, C. L. Using mediation to manage conflict in care facilities. *Nursing Management, 39*(2). Retrieved April 11, 2011, from http://journals.lww.com/nursingmanagement/Fulltext/2008/02000/Using_mediation_to_manage_conflict_in_care.6.aspx

Sullivan, E. J. (1999).Violence and nursing. *Journal of Professional Nursing, 15*(5). Retrieved April 11, 2011, from http://www.eleanorsullivan.com/pdf/violence.pdf

CASE STUDY

Confronting a Bully

Chi chairs her nursing unit's practice council. With her leadership, the council considers changes to improve patient care. Recently, for example, they moved shift report from the nurses' desk to the patient's bedside. The staff felt more involved in the patients' care and safer during shift change, and the response from patients and families was positive.

Chi had one frustration. Often when Chi reported on the council's work during a monthly staff meeting, she noticed that Elaine, another nurse, was rolling her eyes. Once Chi overheard Elaine complain to others that Chi's work on the council was nothing more than "brown-nosing the boss."

Chi debated how to handle the situation. She could ignore it and hope that Elaine's behavior changed—an unlikely outcome. She could confront Elaine privately and ask her to stop her negative behavior. Chi could also confront her publicly, but she decided that would be an ultimate step if nothing else worked.

At the next staff meeting, Elaine again rolled her eyes during Chi's presentation. Chi couldn't allow the situation to continue any longer. She decided to speak to Elaine.

Chi asked Elaine to step into the break room, where they could be alone. "Elaine," Chi said, "I would like to talk to you about a problem. I've noticed you rolling your eyes when I report on our unit's practice council and I've overheard your comments about me 'brown-nosing' the boss."

"No, no," Elaine rushed to say. "I've not done that. You're mistaken."

Chi looked Elaine in the eye. "Regardless, the next time I see this problem, I *will* correct it."

Elaine understood. If she used disparaging remarks or eye rolls, Chi would call her on it. In public.

Elaine kept her disapproval to herself from that point onward.

PART

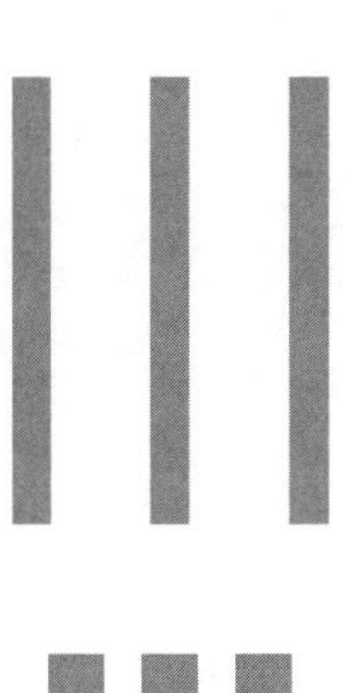

Putting Influence to Work for You

11

Enhancing Your Influence

Don't listen to those who say, "It's not done that way."
Don't listen to those who say, "You're taking too big a chance."
Michelangelo would have painted the Sistine floor,
And it would surely be rubbed out by today.

NEIL SIMON

In this chapter, you will learn:

- How to understand the meaning behind the message
- How to use the finer points of courtesy
- How to handle rudeness and disappointments
- How to take advantage of meetings and travel
- Why persistence, timing, and trust matter
- How to make a commitment to your colleagues now and in the future

ENHANCING YOUR INFLUENCE

People are not alike, and you are not exactly like you were in the past. We're all learning, adapting, growing, and changing. Neil Simon advises us to be willing to learn and grow and change, regardless of what others think or say or do. You won't please all the people all the time, but you don't need to. You need satisfy only yourself.

Continue to assess yourself, reflect on your progress, and seek feedback from others. (See the web resources at the end of this chapter for examples of two assessment tools.) Use people you admire as examples, and think about their actions and behaviors that you can add to your unique personality and situation. Your goal is not to mimic them but rather to learn from them. Some behaviors you will not want to emulate. In fact, you may say to yourself, "That's not how I would do it." That's an excellent way to assess various modes of interacting or managing and discover what will work for you.

INCREASING YOUR SKILLS

If you've been practicing the skills you've learned in the previous ten chapters, you're on your way to building your influence. Like any new skill, influence building requires practice, making mistakes, discovering how to improve, and more practice. Also—like any other skill—you are never finished learning. Each experience is new with that person, situation, or event. The good news is that you never need to feel like it's over and you have failed.

Tomorrow, you have another chance.

For the Novice Nurse

This chapter may read like it's written in a foreign language. But it's not. What's shared here is culled from a lifetime of nurses' experience. It's used by the most influential nurses in the profession and by those who influence via their work at the bedside.

Heed these words well. They'll carry you far.

THE MEANING BEHIND THE MESSAGE

Sometimes people mean exactly what they say. Their words are congruent with their expressions, gestures, and movements. Some people, however, routinely mask their underlying emotions, and most people obscure their feelings at times. Children tend to reveal their emotions even as they say, "I didn't do it."

Most of the time, however, there are myriad meanings behind the words; however, clues to understanding what people really mean by their words is not so difficult. The ability to understand the meaning behind the message is not simple, but it's no mystery (pun intended). Paying attention to nonverbal behaviors such as gestures, facial expressions, posture, and movements is helpful, but understanding what people mean goes beyond noticing these behaviors. It is part observation, part interpretation, and part intuition.

Remember how you learned to observe patients in nursing school? At first, it was overwhelming. How could you be certain to notice everything? Over time, you learned to assess patients' signs and symptoms, quickly noting when something was wrong.

What skills did you use? Clinical observation, certainly. Interpretation of the signs and symptoms, yes. Then you used your finely honed intuition, trained over many experiences, to tell you what to do. Of course, all of this happened very quickly—often instantaneously—with muscle memory propelling you into action.

The same can occur when you learn to read signs that are more ambiguous. We are a verbal society, however, trained to listen to people's words, not to the more obscure signs of attitude, beliefs, and responses. Known as a "tell" in poker, subtext in fiction and film, social intelligence in the social sciences (Goleman, 2007), and by most of us as "people smarts," such signs reveal underlying thoughts and emotions: in other words, what people really mean. It's the "unspoken messages they send by means of their eye contact, the way they move, what they talk about, and what they avoid" (Korgeski, 2010, p. 38).

Watch a movie with the sound muted and notice the actors' facial expressions, gestures, and movements. You'll be surprised how much you understand about the character and the story from such silent observation.

Experts can be trained to observe and interpret micro-expressions, which are fleeting facial changes that reflect underlying emotions—especially emotions the person is attempting to hide (Ekman, 2009a). Trained professionals learn to interpret these minute expressions to discover who's telling the truth and who is not (Ekman, 2009b).

Even computer software can read behaviors and expressions. In one hospital, observant machines watch patients for signs of restlessness or pain (Lohr, 2010). Skilled politicians (or prison guards) can "read" a room the moment they enter it. Police interrogators are experts. So are politicians, salespeople, and possibly even your boss. So how do they do it?

Actually, we all have this ability. It's innate—hard-wired as a survival skill. Even without specialized training, you can learn this skill. It's as simple and as difficult as paying attention.

The same skills that enabled you to recognize patients' conditions will prove useful as you learn to understand what people mean even without having said a word. With practice, you may be surprised by how well you can foster this valued skill.

Start with physical appearance. Is the person's clothing appropriate to the setting? Slacks and jacket are right for business; jeans and a T-shirt are appropriate for casual events. Of course, we've all had the experience of being over- or underdressed on occasion, so consider attire just one aspect of meaning.

Pay attention to how people move, what gestures they make with or without speaking (ever been dismissed with an arm wave?), how they position their body, whether they use touch, their facial expressions, their voice,

BOX 11-1
Examples of Nonverbal Behaviors

- ***Facial expressions***—blinks, curls lips, draws forehead up or down, holds mouth tight
- ***Eye contact***—looks above or below companion, glances away frequently, gazes intently
- ***Body positioning***—stands close, slouches, military posture, relaxes with arms crossed
- ***Movement***—swings arms or legs, taps toes, shifts weight
- ***Gestures accompanying speech***—points fingers, waves arms, holds thumbs up, shrugs
- ***Touch***—self (face, arms, legs, body) or others (hand on arm)
- ***Voice***—tone (harsh?), pitch (high?), volume (soft?), quality (enunciate clearly? slurred?), pace (fast? hesitant?)

and their eye contact or lack of it, among other indicators. Box 11-1 lists some examples. Just remember: these are general indications of emotional content.

Facial expression is the most easily read indication of our feelings, so much so that the term "poker face" is used to describe the ability to mask feelings. Frowns, grimaces, smiles, and surprise often are reflected in the face. Teeth clenched or a hand over the mouth can mean the person doesn't want the words to spill out. Eye contact can indicate interest, boredom, or distraction.

Torso position and posture are the most difficult to read because they are the most easily controlled. In general, open positions signal receptivity and closed positions indicate resistance. Arms across the chest may be shutting out the other person or be protective; cocking the head, leaning forward, and increasing eye contact show interest.

Movement, too, is telling. Few people sit or stand still during conversations. Swinging arms, tapping toes, or shifting weight may indicate resistance. How people use gestures and touch also reveal their feelings. Arms spread wide, hands open or touching the face, and leaning forward indicate interest.

Voice tone, quality, pitch, volume, and cadence are often overlooked in understanding what people mean. Ever tried to hear a person who consistently whispers? What did you do? Lean forward to hear better? Pay closer attention? That may have been his or her purpose.

But here's the caveat: none of these observations are correct all of the time. They're unique to the person, the relationship, and the situation. That's the reason why it's so difficult to interpret other people's meanings. So keep in mind that these are general rules of thumb, not absolutes.

Finally, put together all these observations and interpret their meaning in the context of your relationship and the situation. Ask yourself several questions: what emotion is he experiencing? What does she mean by her words and her actions? Use your experience and your intuition.

This skill takes practice. Try observing people in line at the grocery. Who is impatient? Who is distracted? Walk through your hospital or college and notice the people who pass by. What emotions do you see on their faces, in their movements, and in their gestures? Are they anxious, happy, sad, depressed, or worried? Then try using the skill in your everyday life. See if paying attention to how people speak and behave helps you understand them better.

Such awareness of and reaction to people may sound calculating or false; it is neither. It is simply a process of becoming more and more sensitive to others, enabling you to respond accordingly. Understanding the meaning behind the message is a way to enhance your ability to listen to others with greater perception.

The ability to understand others is useful in caring for patients, responding to patients' families, interacting with coworkers and other health care providers, communicating with people in community or religious groups and professional organizations, as well as enhancing your relationships with friends and family members.

Learn it and be on your way to becoming influential.

BEYOND UNDERSTANDING OTHERS

You've paid your dues in nursing. You've been working for some time in the profession, you've made contacts among colleagues in nursing and other professions, and you've pursued opportunities for advancement. What's next?

People who are influential know more. Also, they can identify other influential people by their use of these subtleties.

The Finer Points of Courtesy

Good manners are invisible. They don't call attention to themselves, and they make others feel comfortable. In addition, courtesy is the hallmark of the influential person. In service-oriented professions such as nursing, good manners are essential (Kahn, 2008).

Pronouncing someone's name correctly and conveying appreciation are two important courtesies. Learn to pronounce people's names, especially if you must use them in public (Pagana, 2010). Joking about how difficult a name is to pronounce is not funny to the person whose name it is. Names of people from other countries and cultures are the most challenging, but they too can be mastered. Solicit help from friends, experts, or the people themselves. They will appreciate such thoughtfulness and remember you for it.

Conveying appreciation is another characteristic essential to becoming influential. A written thank-you note is required after a major event or party, after receiving a gift, or when someone has assisted you in a special way, like introducing you to someone who subsequently hired you. You can use a handwritten note or a written letter, but it must be sent as soon after the event as possible (within a few days, preferably). You can send an e-mail thank-you note if the service was minor and you know the person well. Express your gratitude and add a few comments about how much you appreciate your relationship or friendship.

If in doubt about whether you owe a thank-you note or not, send one. You almost can't thank people too much. (Make a note on your debt list about a favor done for you, and remember that when the person calls in your debt as described in Chapter 2.)

One final mention about courtesy: table manners. Many a position or promotion has been lost over a meal that revealed the candidate's lack of table manners. Knowing every utensil to use isn't necessary, but understanding that adults don't cut up all their food on the plate at once is. See the end-of-chapter web resources for help.

Taking Advantage of Meetings and Travel

Many events offer opportunities to connect with colleagues, learn how others are solving problems, and let other people get to know you. All too often, people fail to take advantage of these opportunities, mostly because they don't know about the possibilities they offer. You learned about networking and making connections in Chapter 8. You can use these skills in local meetings and groups as well as in out-of-town conferences, as shown in the following scenario:

> You go to a professional conference—let's say in another city. You arrive late in the evening after a long day of work, promptly going to your room and ordering dinner in. The next morning you oversleep and arrive late to the first session (missing the continental breakfast) and are forced to sit in the back. When breaks or lunch occur, you sit by yourself because you don't know people there and rush out to make your plane to go home. You may have learned something from the presentations of the day, but you failed to take advantage of many of the opportunities offered.

> Let's see how it could have gone better.

> You arrive at the conference in plenty of time to get settled in your room, register, and review the materials and list of attendees, noting the names of people you especially want to meet and sessions to attend. At the opening reception, you circulate, sharing your card in appropriate circumstances. At the dinner, you find a seat with people you want to talk with or purposely sit with a group you don't know. During dinner, you initiate conversations with your table neighbors, learning about their work and sharing information about yours.
>
> The next day, you continue to network at the breakfast, and when the conference begins, you find a seat somewhere in the center of the room—also next to people you don't yet know. You use the moments before the meeting starts to introduce yourself

to people around you. During the talk, you think of questions you might ask the speaker; if there is an opportunity for questions from the audience, you stand, introduce yourself and mention what institution or organization you represent (do this even if you are not officially representing your employer), and ask your question succinctly. Sit down to listen to the answer. After the speaker finishes, if you have a reason to do so, you make your way to the front and introduce yourself to the speaker, leaving your card if appropriate.

You continue these networking behaviors throughout the conference; on your way home, you make notes about the people you met and any follow-up steps they or you agreed to do. Relax. You've made the most of this opportunity. Next year, when you attend the conference again, review your notes, making sure to connect with selected individuals. You're on your way to becoming influential.

Handling Rudeness

No matter what you do, how tactful you are, or how accomplished you've become, sooner or later (most likely sooner), you will encounter rude comments and behavior. If you're prepared, however, you can counter such behavior with certain tactics. Have you ever been surprised by someone's comments and wished that you had had a snappy comeback? Then thought of one later?

To counter rudeness, you must first understand that you don't have to answer anyone's questions or reply to comments, derogatory or not. No answer is a response. If you simply move on to your topic or another issue, you often can avoid answering rudeness with any statement. Laughing the comment off as if it didn't matter is another way to avoid replying.

Silence, however, is the most powerful response you can use. It is not easy, though, to remain silent in the face of a taunting challenge. Keep your face entirely neutral to use silence most effectively. Most people are uncomfortable with silence and are likely to turn to the perpetrator with blame. You have made your point. Now move on.

Handling Disappointments

It would be great if everything went our way. We got good grades in school, graduated at the top of our class, got the exact job we wanted, and so on. The reality is that few of us get most of what we want—and no one gets it all. Think of the presidential candidate who lost the previous election. Disappointments are a fact of life.

Disappointments can be major ones (e.g., a death, a loss of a job or a relationship) or more minor (e.g., your plane is late). It is important to distinguish between the two and save your grief for those situations that affect your life in the longer term.

How to handle a severe disappointment, such as a death, is beyond the scope of this book, but even seemingly minor losses can cause grief. Allow yourself time to mourn. Confide in people you trust. Know that your grief will eventually pass. Be good to yourself in the meantime.

Sometimes disappointments come from our own regrets. We didn't do what we should have to ensure success (e.g., study for a test). Consider those opportunities to learn what to do or not to do in the future and move on.

There are several ways to reduce disappointments:

- *Ground expectations in reality.*

  Assess the likelihood of success so that if you don't get what you want, you've reduced your level of disappointment.

- *Prioritize your expectations, eliminating those coming from others.*

  Don't think you have to measure up to your parents' or friends' expectations. It's your life; keep it so.

- *Drop a sense of entitlement.*

  Closely related to having unrealistic expectations is thinking that we are owed something just because we're nurses. Drop the idea and concentrate on being valuable because of what you do.

- *Recognize that you can't control everything.*

  You already know this. Remind yourself of it when things don't go your way, and focus on what you can do in the future.

- *Have something in your back pocket.*

  Recall the strategies in Chapter 8 for networking. Keep your contacts informed about what you're doing and stay abreast of opportunities. Have several ideas for the future so that if one doesn't work out, you have another option.

- *Practice resilience.*

  There's only one way to go when you're down, and that's up. Figuratively (or literally, if need be) pick yourself up, dust yourself off, and get going again. Remember: life is a series of ups and downs. Resilience is the secret to overcoming disappointments. Practice it.

Saying "No" Can Be Positive

Commitments are opportunities to learn about leadership, negotiation, and how organizations function and to make new contacts for yourself and your future. Some people agree to anything they are asked, often regretting making the commitment later. Other people tend to say "no" to every opportunity, fearing that they'll be overburdened. Neither tactic will help you become successful.

It is tempting to agree to do something that sounds interesting without considering the effect on our life and career. If you say "yes" but you can't fulfill the task, end up doing a half-way job, or stress yourself unreasonably, you will have let others down and won't have helped your career. On the other hand, being too quick to say "no" might prevent you from pursuing something positive. To decide, consider the following:

- *You won't ever have enough information.*

  No matter how much you learn ahead of time, there will always be surprises. Just make the best decision you can at the time.

- *You can't please everyone.*

  The only person you have to please is yourself. Decide what's right for you in your life, considering your other obligations.

- *You have only so much time.*

  You have the same 24 hours as everyone else. Decide how you want to use them.

- *You must prioritize your obligations.*

  Ask what would benefit the most people over the most time; what would offer the greatest opportunity for learning; what would help your career the most; and finally, what you would enjoy doing.

If you decide to say "no," you know you have made the best decision for yourself at that point in time. And that's a positive for you.

The Importance of Persistence, Timing, and Trust

PERSISTENCE. It has been said that the mark of successful people is not their brilliance, their good looks, or their inheritance. Only one characteristic can be applied to successful people regardless of these other attributes: persistence.

One example of how persistence pays is with education. Being admitted to a school or a program is the first step. Fill out the application, supply the materials requested, take any admittance exams, offer names for references—all this in the time allotted—and you've done the first step. Next, if you show up, participate, and do the work, you have at least a good chance to pass a course and—by doing this course after course—to graduate.

Sounds easy, doesn't it? It isn't. Many people are capable of doing the work and want the degree, but they get tired of going to class or missing fun times. If you are one who does graduate, you've proven the adage. Now apply that persistence to whatever you want to do.

This is not to say that everything you want or try will work. (Remember the importance of taking risks?) Of course it won't. But if you don't try, it definitely will not work. Some things will work out; others won't.

Sometimes life works out better than we've planned. That's a nice surprise. Sometimes we really want to be admitted to a program, get a certain job, be elected to a position in a professional association, and it doesn't happen. Again, maybe something else will occur in our future that will be better. After all, now you're available when that new opportunity arrives.

So what's the secret to being persistent? Habit. We can do almost anything if we make it a habit. This is not easy. Have you ever tried to change your diet, stop smoking, or exercise regularly? How easy was it? But have you become successful with something that wasn't easy in the beginning? If so, you'll realize that you made the change by doing the activity or behavior over and over until it became a habit. Once you make some progress—for example, lose a few pounds—your success helps you keep going. That's persistence.

TIMING. Timing isn't one thing; it's everything, to paraphrase former Green Bay Packers coach Vince Lombardi. What may be right for now may not be right later, and vice versa. Life doesn't work on your timetable. Goals aren't items to be checked off on your "to do" list. Keep timing in mind as you continue to refine your influence skills.

TRUST. Working with people you can trust and being trustworthy yourself is the foundation for influence. There is only one way to earn the trust of others, and that is to be trustworthy. The rule to being trustworthy is: say what you mean, and mean what you say. It sounds simple. It isn't.

Most people tend to avoid saying what they mean out of concern for the other person or concern for the consequences to themselves. This is not to say that you should offer unwanted and unasked-for advice or unsolicited opinions. But don't be obscure, hoping that someone will simply know what you meant or wanted. Others cannot read your mind. So don't hint around; get to the point, simply, calmly, and clearly.

The second part of the rule, "mean what you say," has two meanings. First, it refers to honesty. If you say it, you mean it. Second, it means you agree to follow up and follow through with your obligations, or if for some reason you cannot, you will report that you can't.

Knowing whether you can trust others is more difficult, at least until you have had some experience with them. Pay attention to what others promise and watch to see whether they carry out these commitments. Confront blatant lies, such as the "dirty tricks" mentioned in previous chapters.

Another rule for trust involves using the grapevine. As we've discussed, the grapevine—sometimes called the rumor mill—is a valuable source of information that may not be public. It is, however, seldom accurate. By the time a story is repeated several times, it isn't exactly like the original version, which may or may not have been true in the first place. Nonetheless, the grapevine at times can give you a heads-up, and you can use it to float an idea to see what kind of response you get.

One caveat for using the grapevine: never use it to gossip. Gossip is the spreading of rumors, true or not, about someone's personal life or problems. Gossip helps gossipers feel important because they know something others don't and spreading gossip temporarily raises their self-esteem because they see themselves as better than the object of their gossip. Don't fall into that trap. If other people hear you spreading gossip, they will suspect that you will talk about them as well.

BOX 11-2

Commitment to My Coworkers

As your coworker, with a shared goal of providing excellent nursing care to our patients, I commit to the following:

- I will accept responsibility for establishing and maintaining healthy interpersonal relationships with you and every member of this staff. I will talk to you promptly if I am having a problem with you. The only time I will discuss it with another person is when I need advice or help in deciding how to communicate to you appropriately.
- I will establish and maintain a relationship of functional trust with you and every member of this staff. My relationships with each of you will be equally respectful, regardless of job titles or levels of educational preparation.
- I will not engage in the "3 Bs" (bickering, backbiting, and blaming) and will ask you not to do so either.
- I will not complain about another team member and ask you to not do so either. If I hear you doing so, I will ask you to talk to that person.
- I will accept you as you are today, forgiving past problems, and ask you to do the same with me.
- I will be committed to finding solutions to problems, rather than complaining about them or blaming someone for them, and I ask you to do the same.
- I will affirm your contribution to quality patient care.
- I will remember that neither of us is perfect, and that human errors are opportunities, not for shame or guilt, but for forgiveness and growth.

A Commitment to Your Colleagues

Nurse leader Marie Manthey believes we have a commitment to each other. She suggests that each of us make a commitment to our coworkers and try to follow its principles (shown in Box 11-2) throughout our work life.

ONE FINAL STEP

The last step on the road to influence is your responsibility to return the support you've been given by helping others. Become a mentor, prepare your successors, and leave a legacy. These topics will be covered in the final two chapters in the book.

One more note about paying your dues. As you become involved in other organizations and groups, either in nursing or in other fields, you earn trust and establish your reputation over and over again throughout your career, regardless of your previous experience or achievements. Participate in meetings and offer to serve on committees or in other ways until you become known in the group. Those who try to circumvent this process are seldom influential.

What You Know Now

You now know that you can learn to read others' behaviors by paying close attention to the subtle cues inherent in nonverbal behaviors. You're aware of the importance of courtesy and how to handle rudeness and disappointments without letting either of them get you down. You know how to take advantage of meetings and travel and to help others along the way. You know that persistence, timing, and trustworthiness are essential. You've made a commitment to your colleagues.

Good luck!

Tools for Practicing Influence

1. Practice reading others' behaviors, especially the more obscure or fleeting ones.
2. Take advantage of travel and meeting opportunities to make connections.
3. Learn to handle rudeness and disappointments.
4. Learn the finer points of courtesy.
5. Make a commitment to your colleagues.

Learning Activities

1. Recall a recent interaction that did not go as planned. Describe the other person's nonverbal behaviors moment by moment, such as, "Looked out the window while I talked." What did you do or say? Could you have improved the interaction?
2. Visit a public location where people are seated, such as a hospital waiting room, the lobby of a hotel, or a restaurant. Observe the people around you. See if you can "read" their mood. Are they anxious, happy, sad, depressed, or distracted? Do you see a change after a few minutes? What do you think is going on in their lives? Use your imagination.
3. Make a list of ways you'd like to improve your ability to read others. Tackle easy ways first. Break down your list into small, incremental steps, such as "pay attention to arm movements." Evaluate yourself weekly on your progress.
4. Pay attention to your manners for one week. Note areas that need improvement.

References

Ekman, P. (2009a). *Telling Lies.* New York: W. W. Norton.

Ekman, P. (2009b). *Emotions revealed: Recognizing faces and feelings to improve communication and emotional life* (2nd ed.). New York: Henry Holt.

Goleman, D. (2007). *Social intelligence: The new science of human relationships.* New York: Bantam.

Kahn, M. (2008). Etiquette-based medicine. *New England Journal of Medicine, 358*(19), 1988–1989.

Korgeski, G. (2010). The socially intelligent. *The Writer, 123*(12), 38–39.

Lohr, S. (2010, January 4). Computers that see you and keep watch over you. *The New York Times*, p. A1.

Pagana, K. D. (2010). 7 tips to improve your professional etiquette. *Nursing Management, 41*(5), 45–48.

Web Resources

Emotional and social competency inventory, http://www.haygroup.com/leadershipandtalentondemand/ourproducts/item_details.aspx?itemid=58&type=1

My Skills Profile, http://www.myskillsprofile.com

Marie Manthey's blog, http://mariesnursingsalon.wordpress.com

Post, E. Business etiquette. Retrieved April 18, 2011, from http://www.emilypost.com/business-etiquette

Twibell, R. S., & Thomas, C. M. (2009). Deal with professional disappointment like a pro. *American Nurse Today, 4*(9). Retrieved April 11, 2011, from http://www.americannursetoday.com/Article.aspx?id=6020&fid=6002

Scott, E. S. (2009). Get smart: Increase your emotional intelligence. *American Nurse Today, 4*(7). Retrieved April 18, 2011, from http://www.americannursetoday.com/Article.aspx?id=5814&fid=5792

Print Resources

Goleman, D. (2006). *Emotional intelligence: Why it can matter more than IQ*. New York: Bantam.

Pease, A., & Pease, B. (2004). *The definitive book of body language*. New York: Bantam.

Post, P., & Post, P. (2005). *Emily Post's the etiquette advantage in business: Personal skills for professional success* (2nd ed.). New York: William Morrow.

CASE STUDY

Using Influence Skills

The nursing dean was scheduled to have her first meeting with the university provost since he had hired her. She came well prepared for the meeting. She knew the school's goals for the next year and how those fit into the school's five-year strategic plan. She planned some reallocations and needed some additional funding to expand the nurse practitioner program taught online; she also needed to update the school's network to accommodate this expansion. From her political activities around the state, she knew that some key members of the state legislature wanted the program available statewide.

The provost had risen through the administrative ranks of the university and had powerful allies in the system and in the legislature. He also wanted to help the dean develop into a tough negotiator. He often challenged her in meetings and in person. She understood his strategy, although at times she was taken aback by his directness.

She walked into his office. He asked her and her budget officer to take a seat at his conference table. Already seated was the university's financial officer.

Everyone knew each other. The provost took his time taking off his suit jacket and hanging it on the back of his chair before seating himself at the head of the table.

"Now," he said, smiling at her. "I'm ready to tell you what you can't have."

Without missing a beat, she replied, "And I'm here to tell you how I can make you look good."

The dean got her additional funding.

12

Telling Nursing's Story

Speech is power; speech is to persuade, to convert, to compel.

RALPH WALDO EMERSON

In this chapter, you will learn:

- What nursing's story is
- Why telling nursing's story is important
- How to speak effectively in public
- How to write for the public
- How to tell nursing's story to the media

WHAT IS NURSING'S STORY?

What do you do in the course of a day of work? You may think your work is routine, but could anyone without your education and experience do it? If you knew nothing about nursing and what nurses do, how would you explain your work?

It takes little thought to realize that nursing is a complex set of activities that requires high-level thinking, exceptional skills, and considerable ability to communicate, negotiate, coordinate, and collaborate in order to deliver care. A challenging education is required, and years of experience go into making what is called "a good nurse." Few in society are emotionally, physically, and mentally able to be a nurse.

You are one of those few. Unfortunately, you are also among the few who really know what a nurse does, because nursing's story is seldom told. The lack of public awareness of nursing undermines the work nurses do and restricts nursing's ability to attract young people to the profession. The public, including ourselves and our families, all will need nurses at some time. We want to be sure that nurses are there when we need them, and promoting nursing is one way to interest people in the profession. Nurses, just like other people, want to be proud of the work they do and would benefit from a positive public opinion of nursing.

Strengthening awareness of nursing's role in health care benefits nurses but ultimately can improve the quality of patient care as well. In order for the public to learn more about nursing, nurses must become ambassadors for the profession, speaking in public and to the media. Nurses themselves are the only people who can tell nursing's story.

For the Novice Nurse

You may think you haven't any nursing stories to tell. But you do. Recall your most memorable experience in nursing. Think about it. Then put it into language that the public can understand. See, you have your first story. Think about your second most memorable experience and put it into words to share. And so on.

You're on your way to telling nursing's stories!

TELLING NURSING'S STORY

Why Nurses Don't Tell Their Stories

The effect of nursing's history on today's nurses' silence about their profession was mentioned in Chapter 1. To be self-sacrificing and do what we're told without drawing attention to ourselves was ingrained in nurses' training (yes, it was called training then) in the past.

Just as cultural norms are perpetuated in succeeding ethnic populations, so do nursing's historical norms continue to influence today's population of nurses. Nurses often say, "I only did what any nurse would do," when it wasn't *any* nurse, but one specific nurse who did what he or she determined the patient needed. That care needs to be announced! We cannot hide our lights (talents, skills, actions) under the proverbial bushel. The future of health care demands that nurses explain what they do in terms that the public can understand.

Regrettably, we have not been prepared in our educational programs or in our nursing experiences to promote nursing or—especially—ourselves. Nurses say, "But my satisfaction comes from the work I do, not in talking about it." We think it is enough to do a good job and don't think what we do is anything special. But it isn't. If we don't tell nursing's story, who will?

How Nurses Can Tell Their Stories

Could you describe your actions without using technical language or focusing on the patient's response? For example, instead of "The patient learned . . ." you could say, "I taught the patient . . ." Do you see the difference this makes? In the first example, you give credit to the patient; in the second, you tell what you as a nurse did to elicit the patient's response. The subtle difference between the two statements has considerably more power than is readily apparent. That power rests in the ability to inform the public about nursing's role in patient outcomes. This is no small feat, and one that nurses must consciously cultivate and use.

Journalists Buresh and Gordon (2006) suggest that nurses develop a voice of agency to tell what they do. A voice of agency means using a matter-of-fact manner to state what we do without using jargon, including such words as "manage," "educate," or "coordinate." Every nurse should have three anecdotes of cases to use when asked questions about nursing, they suggest. You can tell about an incident from your work or use examples from others. (Of course, you can't reveal names or any characteristic that might identify the patient.) In response to the perennial question that bright nurses are asked, "Why didn't you become a doctor?" the journalists suggest responding, "If you ask me what I do instead, I can tell you." Use this opportunity to educate your listener about the real world of nursing.

Table 12-1 lists the steps in creating a compelling nursing story.

Here's how one nurse told her story:

> When I walked into Mr. Valley's room, my heart sank to my stomach. I blinked, hoping I wasn't seeing what I was. Mr. Valley was indeed in trouble.
>
> I had only gotten report one hour ago on this man, who'd had a heart catherization with a groin site puncture. I'd talked to him and he said was doing fine. "We are going to have a great night shift together," I told him. He grinned and said, "We better; I got grandkids to get home to tomorrow."
>
> Now he was pale and his eyes had rolled back in his head. I lifted the sheet and there was bright red blood everywhere. I jumped to action. He had a pulse when I checked it, but now it was racing. I hit the staff emergency button and began holding pressure on Mr. Valley's bleeding groin site. His blood pressure was 70/40 and his pulse was raising.

TABLE 12-1 Steps to Creating a Nursing Story

1. Open with a compelling hook.
2. Tell what happened in short, concise, descriptive sentences.
3. Tell what you did in lay language.
4. Close with the outcome that your actions brought about.

> I called out for the unit clerk to call the doctor. Mr. Valley was going to need a transfusion. The doctor arrived and ordered the transfusion.
>
> After an hour, Mr. Valley's blood pressure was back up to 90/68. His pulse had slowed to 110 and he was awake again. He asked if he was okay and said he felt tired. I told him he'd had some bleeding from his groin puncture site, but he was going to be okay.
>
> Mr. Valley said he was glad he had someone taking such great care of him. I was thankful Mr. Valley was going to be okay.

To learn more storytelling tips, watch the YouTube video listed in the Web Resources section at the end of this chapter.

Where to Tell Nursing's Story

There is no end to the places where nurses can tell their stories. Have you ever been at a social event where you've met new people and mentioned that you are a nurse? What happens? Eventually, someone sidles up to you to tell you about his back problems or her mother's increasing forgetfulness or to ask if you can recommend a surgeon. They either ask your advice outright or wait expectantly for some sage opinion from you. At the very least, they are implicitly asking for sympathy, which you are prepared to give though without offering health advice.

This conversational opening gives you an opportunity to tell a story about nursing. You can use one of your anecdotes or a relevant story to talk about what nurses do. It needn't be a long anecdote and most definitely must be told in language the layperson can understand. At least one person will then know more about nursing than he or she did before—and who knows how many opportunities in the future that person will have to pass your story along.

Your family members are excellent people to whom you can tell your stories. You have the advantage of talking to people who care about you. Just think of the number of people each member of your family might be able to tell others about nursing's work thereafter.

Community organizations, religious programs, PTA meetings, and service organizations all need speakers; at such gatherings, you can give a more formal presentation, and these situations offer opportunities for informal chats as well. Take advantage of any of them. You never know when you will meet someone who will influence others' opinion about nursing or interest someone in entering the profession. In addition, some of these people are likely contacts for your network and may help you develop in your career. (More about career planning in the next chapter.)

Never forget that everywhere you go, you represent nurses and the nursing profession. Let your attitude and your words tell the world how nursing is an indispensable component of health care.

TELLING NURSING'S STORY TO THE PUBLIC

Speaking in Public

Some people make a career of public speaking. Most of us, though, are called upon to speak in public as part of our role in an organization. A nurse who works on the burn unit at a pediatric hospital might be asked to teach fire safety at an elementary school. An oncology nurse might talk to a women's group about breast cancer. A nursing school's recruiter might address a group of high school counselors. Each of these opportunities offers a chance to enlighten and inform audiences about nursing.

Speaking in public, however, is seldom anticipated with delight. Those who are not career speakers (most of us) can nonetheless become confident, skilled presenters with preparation and practice.

PREPARING YOUR TALK. *First, decide the purpose of your talk.* Is it to inform, persuade, move to action, or all of the above? Dana, whose story is told in this chapter's case study, wanted to inform junior college students about the opportunities and satisfactions of being a nurse.

Second, what do you want your audience to do as a result of your talk? Speaking to a group of parents, you might want to teach them about fire safety in the home or persuade them that vaccines are safe for their children. Dana hoped to persuade some of the students to apply to nursing school.

Third, what are your three main points? Dana listed hers. They were:

1. The demand for nurses is increasing and is expected to continue to do so.
2. Nursing offers career-long opportunities.
3. Nursing is an interesting, satisfying, and rewarding career.

Fourth, create an outline. Don't groan. It's not an outline that anyone will see or grade. Just list a few words about your opening, the three main points, what action you want your audience to take, and your conclusion. Leave plenty of space between topics for the following step.

Fifth, add notes for your talk. Under each topic, jot down a few notes on the subject. Don't worry if you can't fill in all the blanks. You are just beginning the process now. Take some time to brainstorm, jotting down ideas, phrases, or single words as they come to you without trying to evaluate them.

Use stories and examples to illustrate your main points. Make other people the hero, not you. Give credit to your mentors or people whose examples you follow. Dana told the story of her grandmother's nurse, and she injected the example of the critical care nurse who influenced her decision to work in intensive care. Also, tell about situations you faced and what you learned from them. Be specific.

Step away from your notes for some time and come back to them when you have an opportunity, but keep the talk in your mind. You may have bursts of creative ideas when you least expect it. This time for incubation is essential. Don't expect to sit down and write out a talk in one sitting. You and your talk will be the poorer for it.

Finally, you are ready to prepare your talk. In some instances, a presenter wants a speech written out in full. If you are presenting a formal report or speaking to a large audience or are new to giving speeches, you may want to be able to read from a printed copy of your speech. If you do, you must practice, practice, practice so that you can speak directly to the audience. Nothing is more deadly than listening to someone reading a speech, head buried in the paper, regardless of how compelling the content is.

Accomplished speakers prepare their speeches in outline format using key phrases, sentences, or notes. Some write out completely the first few sentences to help get them started as well as a few concluding statements so that they are certain to include them. Practicing is essential in this case as well because you must be thoroughly familiar with your material in order to deliver it smoothly and professionally. Regardless of whether you write out your speech or use notes, practice until you feel comfortable with the content and are certain what you want your audience to know and do.

HOW TO PRACTICE. Giving a talk is more than sharing information, no matter how interesting it might be. Your voice tone, pitch, and pace, coupled with your posture, gestures, movements, facial expressions, and eye contact all affect how well your talk is received.

Record yourself on video or audio after you've practiced and think it's ready. Play it back and you'll likely be surprised how you look and sound. Maybe you drop words at the end of a sentence. Or shuffle papers. Or talk too fast. Or slow.

Now is the time to make changes, rehearse, and record again. Keep practicing and recording until you're satisfied with the result. By that time, you should also be comfortable with the content, but don't hesitate to change a few words when a better word comes to mind.

GIVING THE SPEECH. No matter how much you have prepared, when it comes time to speak, even experienced presenters have a few jitters. Adequate preparation and practice help, as described previously. Once you begin to speak, you'll find that your nervousness diminishes.

Focus on the audience. It's best to circulate with attendees before the talk. You become more comfortable because you can relate to people as individuals, and they will warm to you.

Review your posture, movements, expressions, and gestures once again, and after you're introduced, step out confidently. You have much to share, and they are ready to listen.

Be prepared for questions, both formally in the session and afterward. Use this opportunity to support other people and possibly to expand your network and theirs.

One note of caution for experienced speakers: even though you may have given the talk to other audiences, the people in front of you have not heard it, and they deserve the same enthusiasm and attention you gave to your first audience. Remember to also speak the language of the audience, which requires you to learn as much as you can before you prepare your speech or—at the very least—prior to your presentation. You want the audience to identify with you and for your words to resonate with them. Using their language and referring to examples they find relevant can help ensure such an audience reaction.

Writing for the Public

Heinrich (2009) suggests that mixed messages about writing permeate nursing. Other professions foster publishing, considering it a professional obligation. Nurses, however, are often discouraged, not wanting to call attention to themselves or be criticized for "blowing their own horn."

Individually, nurses must overcome their reluctance to tell their stories, and nurses must collectively support the efforts of other nurses to promote nursing. Only then will nursing take its rightful place in the public eye.

Avenues for nurses to communicate with the public exist in popular publications. Newspapers offer opportunities for opinion-editorial essays, known as op-ed pieces (see "Writing an Op-Ed Commentary on Nursing" in the Web Resources section at the end of the chapter for the link). Nurses can also contribute letters to the editor and book reviews; magazines have sections for nonprofessional writers as well. Community organizations and newspapers often seek opinion-based and informational essays and articles.

Nurses are appropriate authors for many of these publications because of their knowledge and experience in health care as well as their participation in community activities (Smith, 2010). Nurses' perspectives are often different than the viewpoints of professional writers or those offered by other professions. For example, physicians or hospital administrators may have quite different opinions about the nursing shortage than nurses. Nurses' voices can be heard only if nurses themselves participate in the public arena.

Often nurses (and others) are reluctant to contact newspaper or magazine editors because they are not professional journalists. In reality, journalists have a lot of space to fill online or in print on a daily or weekly basis. (More about contacting the media later in the section "Telling Nursing's Story to the Media.")

A few cautions, however. Contact editors only when what you have to say is relevant and you have verified your facts. Be sure that what you have written is the best you can do, and if you are an inexperienced writer, have someone with greater writing skill review your work and advise you regarding the focus and persuasiveness of your message as well as sentence structure and grammar, if necessary. In fact, it is always advisable to let someone else review your writing because even experienced writers can miss important points when they are too close to the subject to be objective.

Another avenue for nurses to be heard is on radio or television call-in programs. With multiple stations and channels hosting guests discussing a wide variety of topics, including health care, nurses have ample opportunity to lend their voices to discussion and debates relevant to them. Again, these programs depend on audience participation and welcome responses from listeners.

Reluctance to appear foolish—or worse—often inhibits people from participating in these public forums. Also, they recognize that selections for national publications are highly competitive. Remember what the admissions counselor told a student about his hesitancy in applying to graduate school: "If you don't apply, I can guarantee you won't be admitted." By the same token, if nurses don't speak out for themselves and their profession, their voices won't be heard.

SPEAKING AND WRITING FOR NURSING AND HEALTH CARE AUDIENCES

You may also have opportunities to communicate with nurses and other health care professionals in public forums. Opportunities include articles, book chapters, columns, or guest editorials in professional journals and books and presentations at professional meetings. Here, again, you can tell nursing's story. Speaking to other nurses, you have the opportunity to share your experiences, inspire renewed hope in the profession, and motivate other nurses to become involved in promoting nursing. Speaking to other health care professionals, you can provide an accurate picture of the vital work nurses do, inspiring new appreciation for nursing's contribution to health care.

TELLING NURSING'S STORY TO THE MEDIA

You learned in Chapter 4 that nursing is seldom mentioned in media reports of health care. This lack, of course, reflects the absence of nursing in the public eye. Changing nursing's invisibility is one of the goals of this book.

Nurses are often surprised to learn that they have newsworthy stories to tell. For several reasons, nurses' stories can be news. Nurses work in exciting and challenging environments and care for patients in complex and compelling situations. Because everyone will eventually need a nurse, these events are of interest to the public, and thus the media are interested. Nursing research, advances in patient care, and nursing's invaluable role in patient recovery are all potential topics for the media.

Members of the media report, though, that nurses seldom are willing to talk to them *even when they are asked*! Reporters commonly hear, "You'll have to talk to the doctor/administrator about that" in response to their requests for information, even when the topic involves nursing. Sometimes nurses decline to speak to the media, citing the press of time. "I'm too busy right now" or "I'll get back to you next week when I have more time" are responses that reporters also hear to their queries about nurse researchers' work. These nurses fail to understand the deadlines that constrain the media. Usually only a short period of time—often a few hours—can elapse until a story is due for a newspaper, website, television, or radio news. Nurses who want to tell their stories must be ready to respond to media requests at a moment's notice.

Nurses often believe that they need their employer's approval to talk to the media, regardless of the topic. Nurses, like anyone, can speak to the media without their employer's authorization, as long as they don't identify the employer by name or other means (e.g., as a local psychiatric hospital when there is only one in the community). "RN" designates a nurse's credibility and is all that is needed for a nurse to respond to the media if the nurse is an expert or has information about the topic. Postoperative care of a heart transplant patient is an example. If, however, nurses are representing their institution, they must work through the appropriate channels in the organization before speaking to the media. Usually this involves the organization's public affairs offices (also called public information or public relations).

Few public affairs officers are familiar with nurses' work, and fewer still think to call on nurses when the media request information. This is as true of nursing schools in universities as it is in nursing units in health care organizations. Helping public relations staff and health care administrators understand the vital role nurses play in patients' recovery and getting them to call on nurses as well as physicians is a major task in the goal to become influential.

> One medical center publication featured an article on a new pediatric unit about to be opened. The accompanying photo showed a clinical nurse specialist putting together children's play equipment, but unfortunately, the equipment and the nurse were positioned in such a way that it looked like the nurse was cleaning the floor.
>
> But that wasn't the worst news. When the nursing administrator brought the photo to hospital administrators and public relations staff, they saw nothing wrong with the picture! They had no awareness that such a photo, though not derogatory, did nothing to portray the actual value that the pediatric nurse specialist brought to the unit—a potential major marketing tool for the hospital.

What do you need to do to contact the media? Two relationships are key to your ability to interact with the media. One is the internal public affairs staff in your institution. Unless they know what nurses do and what expertise nurses can offer the media, these staff members will continue to ignore nursing expertise when they receive media requests. Similar to effective political lobbying (see Chapter 6), getting to know people *before* you need them can lead to them thinking of you in the future. For example, if your public relations staff know that you and your nurse colleagues are experts on the burn care of patients, for example, they are more apt to call you when a disastrous fire has placed several patients in the burn unit.

Next, establish similar relationships with the external media, if possible. The same rules apply as with the internal staff. A reporter might call you on a story that he or she is preparing on fire safety, for example, because you had described the fire prevention program you present at local schools when you met the reporter or responded to a news story. News outlets encourage contact with the public because it gives them visibility and access to news sources.

Think of working with the media as the way you can help them do their job. They have to fill space online, in print, or in on-air time regularly. You can help them with suggestions for stories, innovations in patient care, reports of nursing research, and stories of nurses doing unique work, to name a few opportunities to promote nursing to the media.

What You Know Now

You have learned that nurses have often been silent about their contributions to patients' recovery for a variety of reasons. You know that nurses must overcome their reluctance to tell their stories in order to rectify misconceptions about nursing and recruit future nurses. You have learned ways that nurses can learn to tell their stories and how nurses can be prepared with anecdotes about nursing care. You have learned strategies for speaking and writing about nursing. Finally, you know how and when to approach the media.

You are ready to tell nursing's story!

Tools for Telling Nursing's Story

1. Consciously develop your own belief that nursing is essential to the health care system. Emphasize that conviction with your colleagues.
2. At every opportunity, be willing to tell the public and the media what nurses do and how nursing care affects health and recovery.
3. Collect three anecdotes about your work and be prepared to share them with others.
4. Let both internal and external media know that you are willing to speak to health care audiences, public groups, and the media about nursing.

Learning Activities

1. Using the ideas you developed in the Chapter 4 activities, prepare a communication plan or develop a new plan based on a timely topic. If appropriate, write a letter to the editor or an op-ed piece or contact your local media directly.
2. Following the guidelines suggested in this chapter, prepare a speech about nursing. Use your anecdotes to explain the work you do. Be ready to adapt your

speech to a specific audience. Now, look for an opportunity to give your speech. Or join Toastmasters International.

3. Either record your speech beforehand or, when you give it, ask a friend in the audience to give you honest feedback on your performance. Use this feedback to improve your next presentation. Look for another place to give your talk and evaluate yourself again. Continue this process over time, improving as you do.

References

Buresh, B., & Gordon, S. (2006). *From silence to voice: What nurses know and must communicate to the public* (2nd ed.). Ithaca, NY: Cornell University Press.

Heinrich, K. T. (2009). Why more nurses should write for publication (but don't). *American Nurse Today, 4*(8), 11–12.

Smith, L. S. (2010). Good news about writing for your local paper. *Nursing Management, 41*(5), 43–46.

Web Resources

Sullivan, E. J. (2000). Speaking up; Speaking out. *Journal of Professional Nursing,* 16(2). http://www.eleanorsullivan.com/pdf/speaking.pdf

Sullivan, E. J. (2001). Writing an op-ed commentary on nursing. *Journal of Professional Nursing, 17*(1). http://www.eleanorsullivan.com/pdf/commentary.pdf

YouTube videos: NPR's Scott Simon: How to tell a story. http://www.youtube.com/watch?v=tiX_WNdJu6w

Cardillo, D. Learn to speak with style for fun and profit. http://www.dcardillo.com/career_tape.html

The Teaching Company courses, available at public libraries and at http://www.thegreatcourses.com/greatcourses.aspx

Analysis and critique: How to engage and write about anything. http://www.thegreatcourses.com/tgc/courses/course_detail.aspx?cid=2133

Art of public speaking: Lessons from the greatest speeches in history. http://www.thegreatcourses.com/tgc/courses/course_detail.aspx?cid=2031

Additional Resource

To become an experienced public speaker, consider joining Toastmasters International, where you can speak publicly in a safe and supportive environment. More than 8,900 chapters meet weekly in nearly every city. See http://www.toastmasters.org for information.

CASE STUDY

Telling Nursing's Story

Dana had worked as a nurse for 12 years in several different clinical areas. Dana's friend, Susan, a teacher at the local junior college, asked Dana to speak at a career fair for junior college students considering various career options. Dana loved her work and was excited to share her enthusiasm about nursing. She knew that it was her job as a nurse to champion the importance of nursing and the work nurses do. She also wanted to encourage new people to explore the profession of nursing.

Dana prepared for her ten-minute talk. She thought about the students and what they might want to know. Then she planned her opening, decided on her three main points, and determined how she would end the talk. She practiced the talk, using an outline form of notes because she knew the topic so well.

When the day came for her to present, Dana entered the room with some trepidation. There were more than 50 people in attendance! Nevertheless, she squared her shoulders, took a deep breath and smiled at the audience.

They returned her smile, and she launched into her favorite topic: "I became a nurse because I saw my grandmother cared for by an excellent home-care nurse. I could see how satisfying it would be to know that you're helping people when they need you the most."

After her talk she offered to answer questions. "So what's your career been like?" a young woman in the front row asked.

"I thought I wanted home care, like my grandmother's nurse, but when I started a rotation in intensive care, I met this most amazing critical care nurse, and I knew where I wanted to work. I've loved every minute of it."

"Well," the young woman asked, "why not become a doctor?"

"I thought about that. But I learned that doctors deal with disease and trauma; nurses treat the whole person. Besides, we're with patients for hours, compared with their minutes with the doctor."

"What if you want to advance?" the woman asked again.

"There are lots of opportunities to advance in the clinical setting. I might apply for a management position in the future. Also, there are many positions outside of the hospital in clinics or home care, or you could pursue research or teaching. Pharmaceutical and insurance companies hire nurses. You could become a nurse lawyer, a consultant, or a case manager. You are limited only by your desires."

Afterward students clustered around Dana to ask more questions. She offered them her e-mail address, telling them to feel free to contact her if she could answer questions or help them.

Walking to her car, Dana thought about how well her talk had gone. She smiled to herself.

13

Managing Your Career

If you don't know where you're going, any road will get you there.

L. Frank Baum, *The Wizard of Oz*

In this chapter, you will learn:

- Why you need to manage your career
- How to obtain your first job
- How to build your career
- How to select educational programs
- How to find and use mentors
- How to keep your career on track

WHY MANAGE YOUR CAREER

Nursing is more than a job; it's a career in a profession that offers an opportunity to serve others. Nursing can be a rewarding and satisfying career, but too few of us think of managing our career in nursing (Federwisch, 2010). For the most part, we consider job opportunities as they appear, with little thought of planning ahead to meet our personal and professional goals.

You have many years to work; don't leave your career to chance (Borgatti, 2007). You can plan and manage each step of the way in your career, keeping focused on your goals and pursuing the best routes to meet those goals. This way, each job can teach you, and every experience can contribute to your learning. By planning your career, you can identify what experiences, education, and contacts you need. A plan helps keep your career on track.

THE DIFFERENCE BETWEEN A JOB AND A CAREER

A job and a career are not just different words for the same phenomena. A career is much more than a job, although a job offers an opportunity to make a contribution and to serve others, the reasons nurses often give to going into nursing. A job is a contract between you and an employer; a career is a planned commitment to yourself. (See Table 13-1.) A career consists of a series of jobs, education, experiences, contacts, and obligations that together create a consistent pattern of opportunities to meet your goals. A career is based on your own particular interests, desires, values, and personality matched with opportunities for employment, professional organizational work, and your lifestyle. A career offers a lifetime of satisfaction.

For the Novice Nurse

Finally, a chapter especially for you. From applying for your first job, interviewing, and accepting the position, you know what you need to begin your career in nursing. Beyond your initial job, you can create a great résumé, determine your learning needs, find and work with mentors, and know what to do when life takes an unplanned turn.

You are ready for a great career!

CHOOSING YOUR FIRST JOB

The first step after you've completed your basic nursing education is to select your first job. The purpose of this job is to learn as much as you can and to

TABLE 13-1 The Differences Between a Job and a Career

Job	Career
Contract between you and employer	Commitment you make to yourself
Reactive	Proactive
Other-directed	Self-directed
Choice based on immediate needs:	Choice based on long-term goals:
Money	Opportunities to learn
Proximity to home	Chance to network
Schedule	Supportive mentors
Leaving depends on more money or a better schedule	Leaving depends on an opportunity for a better schedule or to further your goals

perfect your clinical skills. Additionally, you will make contacts among your colleagues and supervisors.

Here are some criteria for choosing your first job:

- You will have opportunity to hone your skills in a clinical area of interest.
- You will learn from more experienced clinicians who are willing to teach you.
- The culture of the organization—and especially the administration—are supportive of nursing.
- The organization's mission fits your values, such as a teaching hospital that serves the poor.
- There are opportunities for advancement.

Recognizing that no job is perfect, use the previous criteria to assess a potential position. If the position and the organization fits most of them, especially the criteria most important to you, consider the following additional criteria:

- The schedule fits your lifestyle.
- The institution is near your home.

The least important criteria for selecting your first job is the salary. A small amount more in your hourly pay is worth much less than opportunities to help meet your future goals. Remember, you have a long time to be in your career; don't sacrifice future opportunities for a slight difference in salary now.

Once you have applied for a position and the organization contacts you to say that they are interested in meeting you, you will agree on a time and place for an interview. The interview is your chance (sometimes your only chance) to sell yourself to a potential employer. Make no mistake: if you can't sell yourself, no one can. You need to prepare for your interview just as you would for any other important meeting. That includes knowing who you are meeting, learning as much as you can about the organization, and anticipating questions you might be asked.

INTERVIEW SAVVY

The Organization

Ask for the name or names of the people who will be interviewing you and for their positions and roles in the organization. Typically, you'll be interviewed by someone in the human resources office as well as the person who would be your supervisor. Possibly, you'll have a joint interview with several people in the organization. Find out their names and positions.

Be especially courteous to office staff; they have the power to smooth your way or report your behavior to their boss. Try to schedule your interview for a time when you can be rested and unhurried, not right after a long day at work or when you must be somewhere else immediately afterward.

You've probably studied the information about the organization online, and you will probably be sent some information about the organization as well. A position description is essential. You can use it to compare to your qualifications. Also, the organization's mission statement, vision for the future, and goals might be included either online or in materials sent to you. Expect to see only the best. You can find out more in the interview.

An organizational chart also is helpful but not always available. The important information for you is where this position fits in the organizational structure, which tells you to whom you would report and that person's reporting relationship. The most direct line to the top administration is the most powerful.

What to Wear

Most people anguish over what to wear to an interview . . . with good reason. The way you dress creates your first impression and can enhance or detract from your words. Keep it simple and conservative. You want the interviewer to focus on your qualifications, not your clothing.

Clean, pressed slacks and tie and jacket for men are appropriate. Women can wear a pantsuit or a skirt or slacks, blouse, and jacket in neutral colors with low-heeled shoes, neutral hose, and simple jewelry and handbag or briefcase. Wear something you feel comfortable in and resist the urge to buy a new outfit unless you don't have anything suitable in your wardrobe. (Refer to Chapter 4 for some more image-related ideas.)

Preparing for the Interview

The purpose of an interview is twofold: for a potential employer to learn about you and for you to learn about the organization (Krischke, 2010). Ideally, the two of you will discover whether there is a role for you in the organization—what is known as a good "fit."

To prepare for the interview itself, identify:

- What you want to know about the position and the organization.
- What questions you might be asked about your education or past experiences. Be prepared to describe your achievements briefly.
- What you think your strengths and weaknesses are and how those fit with your potential employer's needs.
- What you want to know about the organization and the job.

For the interview, take along a copy of your résumé in case yours is misplaced. Also, you can refer to it if you are asked to explain an item. Get explicit directions to the building and office where you will go and plan to arrive a few minutes early. Get yourself mentally ready by reminding yourself of the qualifications you bring to the position and noting items on the position description that fit you.

Enter the office with confidence, smile, and shake hands firmly. Some small talk will ease the two of you into the interview itself. (See Chapter 8 for more about small talk.)

TABLE 13-2 Examples of Interview Questions

Your Current Job
What do you do in your present job?
What do you like best about your present job?
What do you like least?
Why do you want to leave your present job?
Your Achievements and Goals
What are you most proud of accomplishing?
What do you think you do especially well?
What are your areas of weakness?
What are your long-term goals?
What do you plan to do to meet your goals?
Your Interest in the Position
Why are you interested in this position?
What do you see yourself doing next?
Why do you think you are right for this position?
Is there anything you would like to add about your qualifications that we haven't already discussed?

Table 13-2 lists examples of questions you might be asked in an interview in addition to questions about your education and work history. Answer questions honestly, but don't feel that you must explain anything you are not asked. You will have an opportunity to ask your questions about the position and the organization; be sure you are prepared to do so. A candidate without questions implies a lack of interest or expertise.

Most interviewers today understand what questions are and are not legal to ask. You are not required to answer questions about how many children you have, their ages, or your marital status, for example. Just being asked such questions indicates an organizational bias, and you might want to think again about your interest in the organization.

After the Interview

Send a post-interview thank-you letter within 24 hours of the interview to everyone who interviewed you. Your letter can be handwritten on good-quality notepaper or typed on letter-sized paper. It should be brief, thanking the interviewer for his or her interest in you and saying that you enjoyed the meeting. Include a few words summing up your qualifications that fit the position and end by saying that you are looking forward to hearing from them soon.

A Second Interview

It is not unusual to have a second interview if you have passed initial scrutiny and appear to be an appropriate candidate for the position. The second interview usually includes colleagues and managers with whom you will work. You will probably tour the unit and meet potential coworkers, giving you an opportunity to assess the environment.

Situational questions are often asked at this time. For example, you might be given a scenario and asked how you would handle the situation. Take your time to think through an answer. Obviously, they think you can handle such situations because you were offered a second interview. Keep your answer short and to the point. Your goal is to show that you are a competent, confident professional.

This is also your opportunity to find out what you want to know about the specific responsibilities and challenges of the position. You might ask, "What are the most pressing problems facing the unit?" or "What do you need most from a nurse practitioner in this clinic?"

You will probably be asked whether you are still interested in the position; if you are, ask when a hiring decision will be made. Following this interview, again send thank-you letters, but only to the new people who have interviewed you.

Accepting the Position

When you are offered the position, you have an opportunity to negotiate. Don't ignore this chance in your excitement of getting the job.

Salary is usually the main topic for negotiation. Most employers have some flexibility with salary if they have a justifiable reason for it, but they will seldom tell you that. It is much more common to offer the lowest salary they can and see if the candidate asks for more. Ask for more than you would accept, but don't get carried away. Asking for a salary way above comparable amounts is not only unprofessional but also makes you appear to be more interested in the money than the job. (See Chapter 9 for more information on negotiation.)

You can negotiate regarding scheduling as well, as long as it doesn't make your schedule too different from others in similar positions. You might also negotiate for other perks, such as a parking place or vacation days, but acquiring those are unlikely unless others have them too. Management cannot appear to give you more perks than those of other employees who have been with them longer. You want to start your new job on an even footing with coworkers.

Follow up your verbal agreement accepting the position with a formal letter of acceptance to the administrator who hired you. Thank the individual for having confidence in you and your potential, and state again how pleased you are to be joining the organization.

Declining the Job

Sometimes you will decide to not accept a position offered to you. It might not be the right job, at the right time, or in the right organization. Be sure to let the appropriate person know as soon as possible. Thank them for the offer and the confidence they have in you. Explain briefly why you cannot accept at this time and state that you hope they will keep you in mind in the future. Follow up with a letter as well. Even if you are not interested in this position or this organization, someone there might prove valuable in referring another organization to you in the future, for example. Your career will be long; never alienate potential connections.

BUILDING A RÉSUMÉ

Now is the time to keep track of everything you are doing so that when the time comes to apply for a new position, you are not frantically trying to remember your accomplishments, what continuing education programs you took, or when you completed the course at your hospital. Keep a log of your activities. Note the name of the program, activity, certification, or accomplishments; add the dates, who sponsored it, and where; and note anything special you received or learned. Include a list of accomplishments on your job, such as teaching a class or preceptoring students, or skills you've acquired. Table 13-3 offers an example of a format you could use.

Not every item on your activity log will go on every résumé. Résumés must be crafted to meet specific submission purposes. For example, the résumé you submit to an organization to be considered for membership differs from one you would use to apply to graduate school. Having a comprehensive list of all your activities and accomplishments helps ensure that when you put together an application or submit your résumé, you will be less likely to forget some of your achievements.

TABLE 13-3 Activity Log for Career Progress

Activity	Content
Education	Include names of schools, location, dates attended, degrees earned
Employment	Include all positions, including summer jobs and part-time or full-time work while in school
Licenses	Include license number and state
Certification/Credentials	Include name, date earned, sponsoring organization
Professional organizations	Include name, date joined, any committees or offices held, with dates
Publications	Include title, name of publication, date
Volunteer activities	Include name of organization and your participation
Accomplishments	Include accomplishments from your job, professional activities, volunteer experiences

Keep track of your expenses as well. Those can be noted in your activity log, in a file, or on a spreadsheet; the information will come in handy at tax time. Keep CE certificates and receipts in a file as well.

Another advantage of keeping a record of your activities is that you can quickly see whether you are meeting your goals. A quick perusal of your list might show you what else you might need to do.

CONSIDERING YOUR NEXT JOB

The time to think about your next job is when you accept the first one. Begin to assess how much you can learn in this job and think about your next step. Take every opportunity you can to learn.

> One new grad had already determined that she wanted to teach nursing but knew that she needed clinical experience before she went on to graduate school. She used each clinical experience as a learning opportunity. She made notes on the patients she cared for and later looked up their conditions, treatments, and meds on her time off from work.
>
> In less than a year, she had compiled a study guide full of her own notes. She began graduate school full-time and continued to work part-time, continuing to add notes throughout her graduate school experience. By the time she graduated, she was an experienced clinician, although the actual hours she spent in clinical work were fewer than most of the other new nurse faculty.

This is also the time to begin to think about what you will need to advance in your career. Evaluate what experiences you need and where you might get those: a continuing education program, on-the-job training, a certificate offered by your institution's education department, or a graduate degree. Is there a license or certification you need? What organizations, such as working at a trauma center or accepting a leadership position in your chapter of Sigma Theta Tau International, could help you achieve your goals? Are there publications or online resources that would help? Nursing blogs or discussion forums can help as well.

There are many ways in which you can prepare for your next job or the next step toward meeting your goals. Regardless of which you choose, you must assess both yourself and the environment.

The first step is to assess yourself. Identify:

- Your personality, values, beliefs, likes, and dislikes
- Your lifestyle
- Your family
- Your friends and social life
- Your hobbies and personal activities
- Your vision of your future

- Your skills
- Your knowledge
- Your nursing preferences

The last item refers to the areas of nursing that suit you best. Do you like a fast-paced environment, such as an ER, OR, or trauma care? Or do you prefer to have time with your patients? Then rehabilitation nursing, a medical floor, or long-term care might suit you better. Which patient conditions and treatments do you prefer? What intrigues you most? Cardiac problems, psychiatric conditions, or diagnostics (e.g., GI lab)? Would you like to work in a clinic, medical office, in home care, or in public health? What about school nursing or occupational health?

This assessment is not done quickly; it involves introspection, asking friends and family members for their thoughts about you, and learning from online groups, reading, or attending programs. It is also flexible and responsive to ways in which you grow and change. How willing you are or might you become to relocate, go into debt, or sacrifice some time to reach your goal? The issues may change over time as your family life or your lifestyle changes.

The next step is to assess the environment. Consider what might change in the health care system with implementation of health care reform. The shortage of primary care physicians and the growth of nurse-managed clinics suggest an increased need for nurse practitioners, for example.

As advances in transplant technology proliferate, new specialties of nurses and physicians are created. Today's noninvasive technology for monitoring and treating patients for a variety of ills and from a distance suggests that many changes in clinical care may be on the horizon.

There are other ways to learn about the environment. Pay attention to popular media reports on scientific breakthroughs and advances in technology. Check professional websites, blogs, and journals or attend programs in your interest area. Joining a professional or specialty organization and receiving their newsletters and publications is especially useful because those target your interests.

New programs initiated suggest more ideas. For example, some schools are preparing clinical nurse leaders in masters' programs or offering a nursing practice degree at the doctoral level (American Association of Colleges of Nursing, 2010). Want to teach nursing? Retirements have thinned the ranks of today's nursing teachers just when more nurses are needed, resulting in a shortage of nursing faculty.

Observing others may prove worthwhile. Many people chose their career path after watching more experienced members of the profession. Nurses who pursue teaching and administration often do so after working with an especially competent role model.

Talking with experts, colleagues, and administrators also is valuable. Keep alert to hearing information, evaluate its credibility, and assess its usefulness to you. This is where your networking skills are helpful (see Chapter 8).

Gathering information is an ongoing process. Your plan will not be fixed; it will change in response to changes in your life, your goals, and the environment.

Nursing offers an incredible array of opportunities in clinical areas as diverse as cardiac surgery and trauma care to home health and rehabilitation nursing. You can be a clinician or a specialist, a teacher, an administrator, or a researcher. You can become an entrepreneur or an information systems specialist, branch into pharmaceutical sales, or, for that matter, write books about nursing—all the while being a nurse.

Consider your plan to be long-term and flexible. No one knows what will happen in our own lives or in the environment over time or what opportunities may emerge. Keep an open mind; talk to other professionals; explore your interests. What we do know is that we are contributing to our own future by what we do today or what we fail to do.

Finding Your Next Job

Because jobs are plentiful in nursing, you have many opportunities for finding the next job in your career. This move must not be taken lightly, however, no matter how many jobs are available. You want to be certain that you are ready to leave your current job, that you have learned and accomplished what you came there to do, that you will not be leaving at a crucial time (e.g., forthcoming Joint Commission visit), and that you have selected the job that fits your needs now. This is a tall order, so undertake it with considerable thought.

There are many ways for you to learn about potential positions. The American Nurses Association offers a Career Center (see the Web Resources section at the end of this chapter) where nurses can search for open positions and post their résumés. If you're interested in a particular organization, go to their website or Facebook page to learn all you can about their mission, their services, and their organizational structure. Try to discern how forward-thinking they are and whether your goals might fit with theirs. This step is where your self-assessment is essential. Once you know what fits you and what your goals are, you are better able to find organizations whose purposes match yours.

Equally as valuable in your job search is your network of contacts. Some of the most desirable jobs are never advertised but are shared with potential candidates by their colleagues. Go through your contact list for people who could potentially help you. Also search for former colleagues or nursing school classmates on Facebook or LinkedIn who might work in areas that interest you. If you find someone who works at an organization that interests you, contact the person. Remember to also help others who contact you.

In addition, career fairs, ads online and in nursing publications as well as faculty from the school where you graduated are additional ways to inquire about opportunities and to let others know you are interested in considering future options.

At this point, it is advisable to keep your exploration low-key and confidential. You don't want your current employer to know that you are considering leaving until you are ready to share that information.

When you are ready to apply for a position, you must make a decision. Some people say that you should alert your supervisor as soon as you apply for a job. If you don't, you're taking a risk that the person will hear about it through the grapevine. On the other hand, you know your supervisor. If you think you'll suffer consequences if you tell your supervisor about applying for another job, you might decide to wait until you see whether you are asked to interview. Your decision also depends on how much confidentiality the future employer can offer. What is absolutely clear is that you must inform your supervisor as soon as you accept a new position.

Leaving Your Present Job

Just as there is a way to finding a job, so too is there a best way to leave a job, says nursing career expert Donna Cardillo (2010). First, check to see how much notice your employer requires. Tell your supervisor immediately, and follow up with a formal letter of resignation. It is a good idea, Cardillo says, to add some friendly comments, regardless of how you feel about the organization, your coworkers, or the supervisor. Your goal is to leave on good terms.

Resist the urge to just walk out, regardless of the situation. The only reason for doing this would be if you are in physical danger and the organization is not providing adequate safety measures—a rare, though not unknown, situation.

Always be polite in your interactions with your coworkers and your supervisor. Resist the urge to belittle the organization or the administration. Negative comments about others reflects mostly on you. Of course, don't say anything that is untrue. If the situation is difficult, the other employees know it as well. You needn't say anything at all, even if you're asked. You never know what the future will bring, and ending relationships politely is best for your future.

ADVANCING IN YOUR CAREER

Your Learning Needs

Pursuing a career involves life-long learning. You can learn in many ways. Formal education, certification, continuing education programs, books, journals, and professional meetings are just a few of the ways you can acquire the knowledge you need.

BACCALAUREATE EDUCATION FOR RNs. Although only half of RNs hold a bachelor's degree today, the Institute of Medicine (2010) recommends that 80 percent of nurses hold the baccalaureate degree by 2020. Most baccalaureate programs in nursing have an option for RNs to complete their degrees without repeating content from their basic program. Many even offer their programs online for busy professionals. (See the American Association of Colleges of Nursing link in the end-of-chapter Web Resources section.)

GRADUATE EDUCATION. Graduate school, in either a masters or doctoral program, offers both didactic content and experience, which might be clinical for a practitioner program or research in a doctoral program, depending on your goals. If you want to be a nurse practitioner, teach nursing, become a nurse researcher, or advance as an administrator, you need graduate education.

Choosing a graduate program is a difficult and time-consuming endeavor. You must learn as much as you can about the program, its requirements, and its graduates' success to determine whether the program will meet your needs. Gather literature, meet with admissions staff and faculty, and talk to students and colleagues. Compare national rankings of the schools that interest you. Request names of recent graduates to contact for references for the program and interview them. Ask advice from your teachers, supervisors, and preceptors.

This is one of the most important decisions you will make in your career. It can also be the most valuable. Take your time, consider your options, and be fully committed before you enroll.

Students often insist that they can't afford graduate school while at the same time buying a new car. They have already made a decision. It's not wrong; it's just a different decision.

A multitude of options are available to pay for graduate school education. Like the decision to select a school and a program, finding sources of funding takes perseverance. The school's financial aid office can help you locate loans and scholarships; service clubs, such as Rotary International, support nursing scholarships.

Knowing your long-term goal helps, especially if you are interested in an area of need. For example, financial help may be available to nurse practitioners who agree to work in disadvantaged areas for a period of time after graduation. The military also offers scholarships in return for a service commitment.

Money for school is not a reason to reject graduate school. Your investment will pay off in the future in both your satisfaction with your work and monetarily. Evaluate what is important for you, not just now but in the future. New cars will always be available, and you'll be better able to afford one after you've finished graduate school and been hired for a higher-paying job.

CERTIFICATION. The American Nurses Credentialing Center (ANCC) is the recognized credentialing organization for nurse certification. More than 80,000 nurses are currently certified by ANCC (2011). Nurse practitioners, clinical nurse specialists, and advanced-level specialties, such as forensic nursing, are offered. ANCC offers test outlines, references, sample questions and answers, review seminars, and online review courses, among other resources to help nurses taking the exam be successful.

CONTINUING EDUCATION. Finding continuing education to further your career is not difficult; determining the quality of the program may be, though. If you receive information about a program that interests you and fits with your career goals, evaluate the information using the following criteria:

- Is the program sponsored by a known organization, such as a college or professional association?
- Who are the speakers? Are their credentials appropriate to their presentations?
- Is the content appropriate to you at this stage in your development—not too advanced or too elementary?
- Can you obtain financial assistance to attend and, if you can, what do you owe the organization? Bringing back a report of a program you've attended is an excellent way to reinforce your own learning, and it gives you an opportunity to speak in public as well.
- Consider attending even if you must pay your own way. You may be able to deduct the expense on your taxes and, after all, you and your career are the beneficiary.
- Can you arrange to be off work, if necessary, and afford the time and expense? Although you should try to fit your schedule around important opportunities, sometimes that is not possible. Don't despair; maybe a better program for you will be offered in the future.

PROFESSIONAL ASSOCIATIONS. Membership in professional associations offers many opportunities for learning. Journals, newsletters, e-mails, conventions, programs, and books are just the beginning. The organizations host annual or biennial conferences with educational components. The opportunity to meet and network with your colleagues and senior people in the profession and to learn by serving on committees, task forces, and boards is immense. Many successful nurses began their career by participating in a professional association.

Nursing associations cover every specialty and interest. Membership in the American Nurses Association is open to every registered nurse through the state nurses association. Sigma Theta Tau International has members in more than 400 chapters who live in 86 countries. Specialty organizations exist for nurses who work in many clinical areas, such as the American Association of Critical Care Nurses or the American Psychiatric Nurses Association. Each of these organizations has divisions, committees, and boards where your time and talents are welcome.

Finding and Using Mentors

One of the most important tasks in your career is to identify and cultivate mentor relationships. A mentor is a person who has more experience than you and is willing to help you progress in your career (Grossman, 2007). A mentor introduces you to key people and tells you what you need to know and do to move ahead. A mentor provides opportunities for learning, counsels you on mistakes, and takes pride in your successes. Much of what is included in this book is the type of information a mentor might share with you.

A mentor may be a senior nurse or in another closely aligned profession who has contacts that can be useful to your career. Often you work for the same organization, but that is not a requirement. You can have more than one mentor—but usually not at one time.

You might identify someone you would like to be your mentor or the mentor might select you. The arrangement of mentor and mentee, however, is rarely named as such. Usually, you find yourself relying more and more on one or two people for advice, or a mentor singles you out for special opportunities or assignments. If any of those do not work out especially well or if the two of you don't seem to be compatible, nothing is lost. You both go on your way without any bad feelings. A person becomes a mentor when positive experiences accumulate, bringing satisfaction to you both.

A number of benefits accrue for both you and your mentor. You gain a sense of accomplishment by working with a mentor, and the mentor acquires fulfillment from contributing to you and—by extension—to your profession. People senior in the field have a responsibility to pass along what they've learned and to prepare those who come after them. These are the satisfactions of a career done well. (See more about preparing your successors and leaving a legacy in Chapters 15 and 16.)

The time will come, however, when you move away from your mentor. You take a new job or your mentor does. Your relationship changes as a result. You may then become colleagues and friends, and you may acquire a new mentor in the new organization. Sometimes you will move ahead of the mentor, a situation that requires tact and commitment from both of you. Accomplished professional people know that they will always owe a debt to their mentor, and they continue to show their appreciation in large and small ways.

KEEPING ON TRACK

When the Plan Fails

Be assured that your plan will not work exactly as you hope (some things might work out better), and you will make mistakes. Remember discussions about risk taking throughout this book? If you don't risk, you won't achieve your goals. So taking a risk means that sometimes you will fail. All influential people have failed. What makes their career progress significant, however, is that they learn from their mistakes and are willing to go on when external events affect their plans.

Taking the Wrong Job

Sometimes you will take a job that is wrong for you. Or your timing may be wrong. Maybe you thought you were ready for a management position, but you were overwhelmed with the responsibility. No job turns out exactly the way we thought it would, but sometimes the disconnect between our expectations and what actually happens is so great that we cannot continue.

Maybe you took the right job but for the wrong reason. You wanted a faster-paced environment and accepted a position in a busy surgical ICU, working nights. You soon discover that the pressure, your loss of sleep, and the acuity of your patients are more than you can handle.

When you think you may have made a mistake, try to get some advice from someone you trust. An advisor, a teacher, or a mentor may be able to help you sort out what's wrong. It may not be the job. Maybe you need a brief period of counseling or to learn better ways to handle stress.

If you decide you must leave this job, do so with as much care as you can. You will undoubtedly be leaving your employer in a difficult position, so you want to do everything you can to help. Also, having short-term employment on your résumé is generally seen as negative, so you want to be able to explain this experience in the future and have your employer able to report that you did all you could to help them once you realized you did not fit the job. When this experience is over, leave it mentally and move on. Ruminating endlessly seldom helps any situation, including this one.

Other events can throw your plan off track. Your spouse is offered a job in another part of the country. You find you're going to become a parent . . . again. Your parents need more care than you have been providing. When events intrude on your plan, you may need to adjust your time schedule, such as taking graduate classes more slowly.

Changing Course

Be aware of your progress and be open to changing course. Your goals will change as your career progresses, as will your ability to assess what fits for you. You may be surprised that you enjoy a particular aspect of your work and decide to pursue a different course than the one you originally intended.

> During her initial psychiatric rotation in nursing school, a student found that she really liked working in this area, especially interacting with patients. In addition, she realized that she had a knack of knowing just the right words to encourage patients to talk to her. Also, she found mental illness intriguing and the various modes of therapy and medications fascinating.
>
> After graduation, the nurse worked on a psychiatric unit before returning to school for a masters degree in mental health nursing, after which she accepted a position in an outpatient clinic, where she served as a consultant on patients' mental health problems to the nursing staff. Yearning to return to direct clinical care, she applied to a doctoral program in clinical psychology, thinking that her excellent grades and her outstanding evaluations would make her competitive.
>
> She was wrong.

She was not accepted into the program. After figuratively picking herself up, she applied to a doctoral program in counseling, a poor second best in her opinion but the only option she thought open to her.

Here is the first lesson you might gain from her experience: it didn't occur to her to consider another clinical psychology program, either in the same city or in another. She assumed that if she was turned down in this program, she would be in the others.

We will never know.

To have a schedule that worked better with her doctoral program, the nurse accepted a part-time position teaching mental health nursing in an associate degree program. And then a strange thing happened: she found out that she loved teaching students! Wondering if her newfound excitement was because teaching was a novel experience for her, she was reluctant to give up her goal of becoming a counselor to consider a career in academia. As time passed, however, she continued to find satisfaction not only in teaching students but also in learning about how courses were developed and programs emerged out of the college's mission and goals. After she participated in the college's accreditation experience, she was hooked on academia.

This was her future—to help prepare the nurses of tomorrow.

A career plan is a work in progress, just like life. We never know what our future will bring. Remain flexible and open. You might discover that new opportunities await you, bringing a better future than one you had imagined.

What You Know Now

You have learned that your career is yours to plan and manage. You know that your career consists of individual jobs, education, accomplishments, activities, and contributions over the years. You have learned how to search for your first job and how to plan for your next step. You have learned how to apply, interview, and accept or decline a position. You have learned how to keep an activity log and build a résumé. You have learned about your choices for advanced education, certification, and continuing education programs. You know how to find and work with mentors. You have learned that you may change course as your career progresses, and you are prepared to take risks because you know that the opportunity for success also carries a chance to make mistakes. You know that you can achieve your goals if you are open to new opportunities and are flexible enough to adapt to change.

Remember: your job is not you and your work is not your whole life. Life is a journey. Enjoy it!

Tools for Managing Your Career

1. Select jobs and professional activities that help build your career.
2. Keep a log of your activities and expenses.
3. Evaluate educational opportunities that fit your learning needs and offer career advancement.
4. Identify and cultivate mentor relationships.
5. Evaluate your career plan periodically and update it with new information or interests.

Learning Activities

1. Begin a career plan. Using the assessment criteria in the chapter, list your attributes and interests.
   Next, make an initial assessment of the environment. You can add to it later as you acquire more information.
   Now, identify two or three career goals.
   Finally, list what you need to advance toward your goals.
2. Build or add to your résumé. Try to add activities and skills you have not considered previously. Jot down everything that comes to mind; you can edit later. Think about what you have accomplished. Give yourself a pat on the back.
3. Assess the effectiveness of the educational programs you've attended in the past. What made them useful to you? What was not so helpful? Use this information to select and evaluate the next meeting or program you attend.
   Think about how you could create a program or make a presentation using the most effective tools you have identified. Make a presentation in class, at a meeting, or at your institution. Or just be prepared to say "yes" when someone asks you to present information about your area of expertise.

References

American Association of Colleges of Nursing (2010). *The clinical nurse leader.* Retrieved online December 16, 2010 at http://www.aacn.nche.edu/cnl/

Borgatti, J. C. (2007). Plan a career, not just a job. *American Nurse Today*, 2(4). Retrieved online November 5, 2010 at http://www.americannursetoday.com/article.aspx?id=6204&fid=6182

Cardillo, D. (2010). Dear Donna FAQs. Retrieved online January 17, 2011 at http://www.dcardillo.com/articles/donna_faqs.html

Federwisch, A. (2010). Strategic moves. *NurseWeek*, 11(2), 22–24.

Grossman, S. C. (2007). *Mentoring in nursing: A dynamic and collaborative process.* New York: Springer.

Institute of Medicine (2010). The future of nursing: Leading change, advancing health. Retrieved online October 15, 2010 at http://www.iom.edu/~/media/Files/Report%20Files/2010/The-Future-of-Nursing/Future%20of%20Nursing%202010%20Report%20Brief%20v2.pdf

Krischke, M. M. (2010). Nursing interview guide, Part II: Asking the right questions at the right time. Retrieved online December 16, 2010 at www.NurseConnect.com

Web Resources

Search for registered nurse résumé templates online for sample résumés.

American Nurses Association Career Center, http://www.nursingworld.org/careercenter

American Nurses Credentialing Center, http://www.nursecredentialing.org

American Nurses Credentialing Center. *The doctor of nursing practice: A report on progress.* Retrieved December 16, 2010, from http://www.aacn.nche.edu/dnp/pdf/DNPForum3-10.pdf

American Nurses Credentialing Center. *The essentials of doctoral education for advanced nursing practice.* Retrieved December 16, 2010, from http://www.aacn.nche.edu/DNP/pdf/Essentials.pdf

Cardillo, Donna. Career alternatives for nurses (3rd ed.). Available in DVD or CD format from http://www.dcardillo.com/career_tape.html

DiLillo, A., Bjurback-Lupinacci, J., & Soroff, L. The rewards of extern-preceptor relationships. *American Nurse Today, 4*(5). Retrieved April 11, 2011, from http://www.americannursetoday.com/Article.aspx?id=5680&fid=5636

Smith, L. S. Resigning without burning your bridges. *Nursing Management, 42*(2). Retrieved April 11, 2011, from http://journals.lww.com/nursingmanagement/Fulltext/2011/02000/Resigning_without_burning_your_bridges.12.aspx

Sherman, R. O., & Murphy, N. The many merits of mentoring. *American Nurse Today, 4*(2). Retrieved April 11, 2011, from http://www.americannursetoday.com/Article.aspx?id=4342&fid=4302

Tuttas, C. A. Waltzing through the behavioral job interview. *American Nurse Today, 6*(1). Retrieved April 1, 2011, from http://www.americannursetoday.com/Article.aspx?id=7398&fid=7360

Print Resource

A list of appropriate and inappropriate preemployment questions can be found in *Effective Leadership and Management in Nursing* (8th ed.), by E. J. Sullivan (2013). The chapter also includes more information about interviewing from an employer's position.

CASE STUDY

Career Planning

As a new graduate, Sienna had successfully passed the state board exam, completed the hospital's orientation program, and started her first job on a psychiatric mental health unit. Every day was different, exciting, and challenging, and this confirmed her desire to become a psychiatric nurse practitioner. Even though she planned to work on the unit for two or three years before considering graduate school, she began looking at the psychiatric nurse practitioner degree tracks at two schools that interested her. Wanting to be certain she had fulfilled any prerequisites prior to applying for enrollment, she compared the programs and met with the admissions' counselors at both schools.

Sienna learned that a psychiatric nurse practitioner, Geneva, worked at her hospital. She asked to have lunch with her. "What challenges do you face?" she asked as they settled their trays on a table by the windows.

The woman took a few moments to add sweetener to her iced tea, then answered, "There are several. The most troublesome is that few nurses or doctors understand mental illness."

Sienna laughed. "I know about that. When I tell people where I work, they say with the 'crazy people.'"

"And I bet they add, 'I could never do that.'"

Sienna agreed. "So, what do you do?"

Geneva sipped her tea. "I keep at it. Each interaction is an opportunity to educate people."

"You seem pretty upbeat about it."

"What's the choice?" Geneva asked, picking up her sandwich. "It's what I do."

"And what I want to do. Any advice?"

"Want a mentor?" Geneva asked.

Her mouth full, Sienna nodded.

"I'd be happy to help. Let's keep in touch." She gave Sienna her card. "Call or text anytime," she said. "And let's have lunch again in a month or so."

Sienna watched her new mentor walk away. Someday, she told herself, I'll do the same for someone else.

14

Balancing Your Life

Don't compromise yourself. You're all you've got.

JANIS JOPLIN

In this chapter, you will learn:

- How to achieve a better balance in your life
- How to separate your personal life from your professional life
- How to create your own board of directors
- How to improve your personal life
- How to take care of yourself

ACHIEVE A BETTER BALANCE

Do you find that no matter how hard you try, you can never keep your life in balance? Either the job is overwhelming or the family is or your private life is or something else throws your equilibrium out of kilter. It's not surprising.

Today the world has changed (Mayo Clinic Staff, 2010). Just a few short years ago, we could answer voice mails and e-mails at the end of the day. No longer. Being immediately available by phone or text is expected, regardless of whether we're at work, on vacation, or asleep. Our lives, it seems, are no longer our own.

No matter how much you want to separate your professional and personal life, aspects of each inevitably spill over onto each other. You're at home and a text comes in about the home care patient you're scheduled to see tomorrow. Of course you must check it. Your schedule might be changed or you might need to gather supplies or something else that might be different from your earlier plans. Or you're at work in a surgical outpatient clinic, ready to scrub, and you receive a call. Your child is sick at school. These interruptions are inevitable.

If you're constantly checking your phone in the car, in the grocery, or even in bed; if you find yourself hurrying to answer work e-mails on off-duty hours; or if you grab your phone to check personal messages between patients, you've sacrificed your freedom to the technology. Stop. Immediately. Begin today to mentally separate the two parts of your life. You are more than your work.

Although caring is the hallmark of the nursing profession, the stress of patient care and system problems can be overwhelming. Stress or compassion fatigue can result (Slavin, 2009; Yoder, 2010). Coping strategies include preventive activities and ongoing support. Newsom (2010) advises nurses to care for themselves so they are able to care for others. Never have we needed to protect ourselves more from constant intrusions for our health, our sanity, and our well-being (Merritt, 2009; Rauh, 2011).

For the Novice Nurse

You've just graduated, passed your state board exams, and accepted your first position as a registered nurse. You are certain your life will now get back to "normal." You won't need help balancing your life now that school's behind you. This is the perfect time, however, for you to consider how to keep your life in balance. Before you become inundated with more and more demands on your time, think through your obligations and what you need for yourself.

You have long career ahead of you; make the most of it!

YOUR PERSONAL LIFE

The first 13 chapters of this book cover professional issues. This chapter is about your personal life. You can bring the same interest and commitment to it as you do to your professional life. The first step is organization.

Create Your Own Board of Directors

Organizations, from corporations to professional associations, have boards of directors. This group of individuals have considerable control over the success of failure of their parent organization. (For more about organizations, see link to "Professional Organizations: How They Work and When They Don't" in the end-of-chapter Web Resources section.)

A personal board of directors is an unofficial group consisting of the people we turn to for advice. In fact, they probably don't even know they are your directors, and you may seldom think of them as such. They probably do not even know each other.

The criteria for selecting directors is their professional knowledge, their interest in you, and most of all, their wisdom. Here are types of people you might consider for your board of directors:

- ***Financial:*** financial planner, investment broker or banker, tax accountant
- ***Legal:*** attorneys for contracts, wills and trusts, plaintiff actions, liability, malpractice
- ***Insurance:*** agents for home, auto, personal liability, professional liability
- ***Medical:*** nurse practitioner or physician for general or specialty care
- ***Personal:*** counselor, psychiatrist, psychologist, social worker
- ***Spiritual:*** religious leader, meditation guide, friend
- ***Career:*** mentors, teachers, senior colleagues

You will undoubtedly have more than one person in a category. For example, you might consult with attorneys who have different areas of expertise, or you might need financial advice from both your tax accountant and your financial planner. You might consult them occasionally, regularly, or periodically.

Just like corporate boards, your directors may change over time as your needs change. Some, on the other hand, may remain long-term directors. There are no set terms of office for them. They may be compensated (e.g., attorney, accountant) or they may find their satisfaction in the relationship they have with you (e.g., friend, mentor). Regardless, their value to you may be priceless.

Keep a handy file of your board member's contact information and remember to use these experts as needed. Go to Learning Activity 2 later in this chapter to learn how to create and use your board of directors.

Next, consider other aspects of your life. These are:

- Physical
- Emotional
- Spiritual
- Intellectual
- Fun

Your Physical Self

You only have one body, and how you treat it, pamper it, or care for it affects how well it will serve you in the future (Amtmann & Amtmann, 2010; Scholar, 2009). This is not news to nurses. But we have a tendency to value others before ourselves. That's what makes us good nurses, after all.

You might say, "It's too late," "I'm overweight," "My back's injured," or—my personal favorite—"I don't have time." But you do. Remember what's urgent and important. Your health is important, and ignored problems can become urgent. Change may come too late.

Enough said. You know what changes to make. Just do it.

Your Emotional Self

Emotional problems can often be overwhelming. Childhood traumas or adult problems can interfere with your work and your ability to enjoy a comfortable and contented life. That needn't be so. Skilled counselors and mental health professionals, as well as self-help groups, are available everywhere. Your employer may offer an employee assistance program.

Even well-adjusted people have occasional problems or chaos in their lives. It's common to be reluctant to share personal problems, but if they are aired in a safe and supportive environment, they lose their power to interfere with your life. If you need temporary help or longer-term support, take advantage of these services.

Your Spiritual Self

You don't need to be religious to have a spiritual life. A spiritual connection helps us deal with suffering and loss, experiences we all have at some time. Spirituality can be as simple as appreciating nature or as complicated as entering a religious order.

Journaling, reflection, meditation, yoga, relaxation techniques, deep breathing, and mindful awareness are just a few of the methods you can use to calm your body, still your mind, and enhance your spirit. (See the end-of-chapter resources for suggestions.)

Only you know what matters for you and what works for you now. What you need in the future might be different. Spirituality is one of the most personal and important aspects of your life.

Your Intellectual Self

"My what?" you ask. "Don't I have enough intellectual challenges at work?" Certainly you do. But most of us develop tunnel vision regarding work. We see what's in front of us and that's all. There's more.

The human brain is built to learn. From an infant's birth until death, we are always learning: how to walk and talk, then how to read, and so on. Just because formal education has ended, learning shouldn't.

Professional articles and programs can motivate and educate us. Nonfiction books (like this one) can enlighten us. Documentaries can illuminate our world, as can travel. Don't stop learning; you're not dead yet.

HAVING FUN

Are you having fun yet? Don't let this chapter or this book discourage you. Having fun is just as essential as eating right and exercising—more so, possibly.

Just like other aspects of your life, what's fun for you may be torture for another. You may love to swim; your friend hates it. Colleagues want to go out for a night of bowling; you can't imagine anything worse. Your neighbor asks you to go to a serious movie with her; you're looking for a comedy. You get the picture (pun intended).

No one, absolutely no one, cares more about you than you do. As caregivers, nurses often believe that taking care of ourselves is not important (Borgatti, 2010). We take care of others, we say, and that's more important. But if you don't take care of yourself, you won't be able to care for others.

Try thinking of yourself as another person needing your care. Treat yourself as gently as you would your sickest patient. What does he or she (you) need right now? Find what brings you pleasure and put that activity on your schedule the same as you enter a dental appointment or schedule a CE program.

Julia Cameron, author of the inspirational book *The Artist's Way* (2002), suggests weekly artist dates. She recommends that a writer or artist schedule a date to go somewhere special alone once a week, advising that this activity can recharge your batteries and provide inspiration to continue your work.

Nurses are artists, too. Our canvas is the care we give, the students we teach, or the units we manage. Our batteries need recharging just as much, if not more, than Cameron's artists.

Try it.

What You Know Now

You have learned that today's world makes it more difficult to balance your work with your personal life. You're aware that technology can control your life and you've vowed to manage it. You've learned how to create your own board of directors. You have explored your personal life, including physical, emotional, spiritual, and intellectual aspects and have learned some ways you might use to take care of yourself. Finally, you've learned that taking time to enjoy your life and have fun is as important as other ways of caring for yourself.

It's your life. Manage it well.

Tools for Balancing Your Life

1. Think about how to separate your personal life from your professional life.
2. Vow to control interruptions, especially from technology.
3. Create your own board of directors.
4. Evaluate aspects of your personal life listed in this chapter.
5. Be persistent about making changes.
6. Take good care of yourself. You're your most important asset.

Learning Activities

1. To create your own board of directors, make a list of all the people you go to for advice and categorize them according to the areas suggested in the chapter. If you have any categories without a director, assess whether you now need or expect to need in the future someone with that expertise. Consider ways to find people to fill those positions, such as asking other directors for advice.

2. Based on the evaluations in the earlier section "Tools for Balancing Life," ask yourself if some areas need improvement. Schedule appointments as needed, such as a physical exam, an appointment with a spiritual advisor, or a mental health checkup. With information in hand, decide on possible changes, make a plan, and follow up.
3. Schedule your first "Artist's Date." Pick somewhere you really enjoy, such as a flea market, hardware store, museum, ball game, dog show, poetry reading, and so forth. Put your "date" on your calendar, and when the time comes, go. Try to relax, think about only the place or event, and immerse yourself in the experience. Notice sounds, sights, and smells. Savor them. Feel yourself becoming renewed. Leave when you feel satisfied and full. Watch how the world feels afterward. Report your experience to a friend or classmate. Schedule your next date.

References

Amtmann, J., & Amtmann, K. (2010). Use it or lose it: Physical fitness for nurses. *American Nurse Today, 5*(7), 45–47.

Borgatti, J. C. (2010). Who are you? *American Nurse Today, 5*(11), 26–27.

Cameron, J. (2002). *The artist's way* (10th ed.). New York: Penguin.

Mayo Clinic staff (2010). *Work-life balance: Tips to reclaim control.* Rochester, MN: Mayo Clinic.

Merritt, C. (2009). *Too busy for your own good.* New York: McGraw-Hill.

Newsom, R. (2010). Compassion fatigue: Nothing left to give. *Nursing Management, 41*(4), 42–45.

Rauh, S. (2011). 5 tips for better work-life balance. Retrieved January 7, 2011, from http://www.webmd.com/balance/guide/5-strategies-for-life-balance

Scholar, G. (2009). Make fitness fit into your daily routine. *American Nurse Today, 4*(1), 31–32.

Slavin, K. E. (2009). Environment, health, & safety. *American Nurse Today, 4*(2), 36.

Yoder, E. A. (2010) Compassion fatigue in nurses. *Applied Nursing Research, 23*(4), 191–197.

Web Resources

Burke, S. Reiki: Ancient healing art for today's new healthcare vision. *American Nurse Today*, 5(3). Retrieved online April 11, 2011 at http://www.americannursetoday.com/Article.aspx?id=6374&fid=6276

Cardillo, D. The write way. Retrieved April 11, 2011, from http://www.dcardillo.com/articles/thewriteway.html

Mindfulness practice downloads. Retrieved April 11, 2011, from http://marc.ucla.edu/body.cfm?id=22

Pelaez, A. Just breathe. *American Nurse Today, 11*(4). Retrieved April 11, 2011, from http://www.americannursetoday.com/Article.aspx?id=6884&fid=6846

Shindle, M. V. Walking the labyrinth: An exercise in self-healing. *American Nurse Today*, 3(8). Retrieved April 11, 2011, from http://www.americannursetoday.com/Article.aspx?id=4090&fid=4042

Sullivan, E. J. Professional organizations: How they work and when they don't. *Journal of Professional Nursing, 17*(4). Retrieved April 2, 2011, from http://www.eleanorsullivan.com/pdf/organizations.pdf

Sullivan, E. J. Renewal. *Journal of Professional Nursing, 19*(1). Retrieved April 2, 2011, from http://www.eleanorsullivan.com/pdf/renewal.pdf

Print Resources

Borgatti, J. C. (2004). *Frazzled, fried . . . finished? A guide to help nurses find balance.* Wesley, MA: Borgatti Communications.

Smalley, S. L., & Windston, D. (2010). *Fully present: The science, art, and practice of mindfulness.* New York: Da Capo Press.

Thornton, M. (2004). *Meditation in a New York minute.* Boulder, CO: Sounds True.

CASE STUDY

Bringing Balance to Life

Sally was a busy nurse in the pediatric unit. She worked a full-time day shift, took graduate classes to become a clinical nurse specialist, had two young children at home, and helped take care of her grandparents. She managed competing priorities and the demands on her time, and she enjoyed the hustle of her daily life. Sometimes, though, the stress of not being able to get everything done threatened to overwhelm her.

Sally knew she needed to find time for herself, time just for her to recharge. She gave herself some time to think about what she enjoyed and what would be realistic given her schedule.

Sally enjoyed reading fiction, especially light-hearted mysteries. She also knew the importance of exercising and wanted to do more exercise in order to take care of her health. Then she made a plan.

Each night she would take 15 minutes at bedtime to relax and read from a mystery before going to sleep. She also decided to allow 45 minutes two days per week when she was off from work and after she had dropped her kids off at school to take a walk outside.

After a few weeks, Sally felt better. The time outside left her with a healthy feeling, and she began brainstorming about how she could work in more time for exercising. She enjoyed reading each night and felt more relaxed at bedtime.

The result of these small changes surprised her. Sally found that she was more productive at work and more even-tempered at home. Most importantly, Sally felt happier and more balanced in her life.

She vowed to continue to take care of herself.

PART

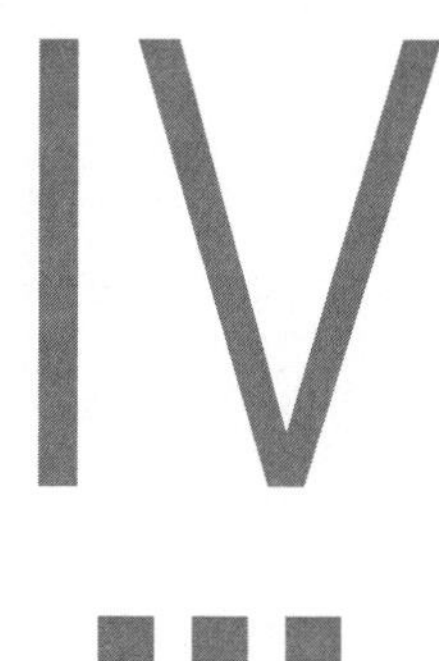

The Final Steps

15

Preparing Your Successors

Vision is the art of seeing the invisible.

Jonathan Swift

In this chapter, you will learn:

- Why you need to prepare your successors
- How to prepare your successors
- How a successor differs from a mentor
- How to become a mentor

YOUR SUCCESSORS

After commencement ceremonies concluded, the dean was greeting new nursing graduates and their families. She asked one new graduate what her plans were for the future, and the student responded boldly, "I'm sorry to tell you this, but I want your job!" Without missing a beat, the dean responded, "Thank goodness. I don't intend to do this forever."

You may think no one can do your job exactly as you do, and you are correct. There comes a time, however, when all of us must move on to another job, another career, or retirement. Face it: you are not indispensable. Before you leave, your job is to prepare your successors.

Your successors are all the people who will come after you, who will take jobs when you finish with them, and who will take other jobs similar to yours. Your successors may be your subordinates today, or your positions may be reversed and you might find yourself reporting to a former subordinate, student, or classmate. Your successors might come from the ranks of your own organization, or they might be professional colleagues working other places. Maintaining relationships, on varying levels of participation, with former students, classmates, colleagues, superiors, and subordinates helps create a cadre of potential candidates to succeed you.

For the Novice Nurse

Preparing your successors is the last thing on your mind. But it should be in your thoughts, because you have the opportunity to be someone's successor! Remember the example of the new nurse at graduation? Both she and the dean knew that she could become the dean's successor. Use this chapter to find mentors for yourself. Someday you'll return the favor to someone else.

PREPARING YOUR SUCCESSORS

Your responsibility to a job or a career does not end when you receive your last paycheck. By then, it's too late to prepare your successors. You should start identifying potential candidates for your position and similar positions and help them prepare for these positions even though you may be reluctant to think about anyone "taking your place."

You will never be finished with a job. There will always be something else you wanted to do, some project that you couldn't accomplish. Recognize that someone else will do "your job" differently; in fact, the circumstances for that person will be different, just as children raised in the same home have different experiences because of their birth order and changes in the family.

Think of leaving a job as an opportunity for someone else. Just because someone does the job differently doesn't negate the value of the work you did. It's just different. The person is different and the situation is different. You contributed your work during your time in the job; now it's someone else's turn.

Preparing your successors gives you the opportunity to pay back the profession for the benefits you've received from others' support. No one among us has succeeded in accomplishing our goals without help from others, even indirectly. All of us craft our career on the shoulders of those who have gone before us. Florence Nightingale began modern nursing, and the many nurses who have followed build on her work. And so it goes, each of us contributing our part to the profession.

Everything you do to share your experiences with up-and-coming professionals—from talking informally to presenting formal papers—helps prepare your successors. Writing editorials or columns in professional publications help prepare your successors, as does consulting with them individually or as a paid consultant to an organization. Writing books about nursing and health care is another way. When you establish programs or teach a class, you are preparing your successors.

When things go wrong, others can learn from your experience, just as you may have learned from others' experiences. Actually, it is rather difficult to not help prepare your successors unless you purposely avoid sharing your experiences with others. Even then, individuals can learn from you just by observing what you do or don't do. Face it: you can't get away from preparing your successors, and that's good. It's the way we learned and the way others will learn from us.

BECOMING A MENTOR

Preparing your successors and being a mentor are not the same, although you may be a mentor to your successor, and in some ways, everyone you mentor is your successor. Mentoring someone involves doing more than helping individuals who may serve after you. Mentoring includes introducing your mentee to influential people and suggesting the mentee's name for appointment to committees or as candidates for office in professional organizations. A mentor is available to counsel and advise the mentee, and usually the relationship is a long-term one that eventually results in a lasting friendship (Grossman, 2007). (See Chapters 2 and 13 for more about mentoring.)

The first step to becoming a mentor is finding people you think have leadership potential. Most commonly, you will encounter such people casually in the course of your work. You will notice that they are competent, enthusiastic, interested in learning, and ambitious enough to be successful. Sometimes they already appear to be leaders among their colleagues, who often turn to them for advice. Of course, few will have all of these characteristics fully developed. That's where you come in.

Your next step is to encourage interaction with your potential mentee. You may be the person's advisor in school or supervisor at work, or you may be colleagues in an organization. You can use informal opportunities, invite the person to join a committee, or suggest the individual for assignments at work or in professional organizations. As the person responds with interest, you continue to advise, counsel, and promote your mentee. Interestingly, you may never verbalize that the two of you are mentor and mentee! Many mentor-mentee relationships are not identified as such.

Your reward comes when your mentee moves into positions of influence. The danger at that point is that when the mentee becomes successful, your influence may be declining as you move into another phase of your life. If you can truly celebrate your mentee's work without jealousy (he or she may have opportunities that you didn't) and your mentee continues to value your assistance, your relationship can become collegial as you continue to support and recognize each other.

So far, we've been talking as if you and your mentee are an independent pair, but that is unlikely. Some institutions have formalized nurse mentoring in their novice nurse orientation programs (Partrick, 2010). Regardless, you will be interested in the careers of several mentees and potential mentees, and they will have more than one person interested in them. There is no limit on these relationships; in fact, multiple such relationships should be encouraged because of the advantage that different perspectives can make in helping a person with a career.

What You Know Now

You have learned that it is inevitable that you will have successors and that part of your job is to help prepare them for their future roles. You have learned that preparing your successors includes all the informal and formal ways to share your experiences and all the work that you have done. You also know that becoming a mentor is not the same as preparing your successors. Being a mentor involves a higher level of involvement in an individual's career and in the person's ultimate success. You have both a responsibility to do so and the opportunity to prepare your successors and be a mentor.

Enjoy the pleasure of continuing to contribute through the work of others.

Tools for Preparing Your Successors

1. Identify people with the potential to follow you.
2. Initiate conversations about their career goals.
3. Discuss preparation for their future.
4. Encourage them to set lofty but realistic goals.
5. Celebrate their successes and support their failures.
6. Maintain an ongoing relationship.

Learning Activities

1. Make a list of everyone who has helped you in your career. Beside each name, list how the person contributed to your learning and your progress. Take several days to do this, especially if you are established in your career. You will undoubtedly think of more people and more examples as you continue to contemplate your experiences.
2. Make another list. On one side of this list, name everyone you have helped in the past, and on the other side, name those you might help in the future. If you are new to nursing, this second list might be short but could include people you knew in school or other organizations. Beside each name, include the activity that helped or might help another.

Compare this list with the one you compiled in the previous activity. Can you add anyone to your list of those you might help? Share both lists with a classmate or colleague.

References

Grossman, S. C. (2007). *Mentoring in nursing: A dynamic and collaborative process.* New York: Springer.

Partrick, D. (2010). Nurse mentoring: Vermont hospital retains new nurses thanks to a nurse mentoring program. Retrieved January 10, 2010, from http://nursing.advanceweb.com/Regional-Articles/Features/Nurse-Mentoring.aspx

Web Resource

Sullivan, E. J. Are we ready for the future? *Journal of Professional Nursing, 18*(6). Retrieved April 15, 2011, from http://www.eleanorsullivan.com/pdf/future.pdf

CASE STUDY

Preparing a Successor

Tyrell was an experienced nurse manager on the orthopedic floor in a hospital near an Army base, a position he'd held for ten years. His long-time partner, an Army nurse, was due to be transferred within the next few years, and Tyrell planned to move with him. Fortunately, Tyrell's mentor had taught him that his job included preparing his successors.

Tyrell scheduled a meeting with the chief nurse, Sharisse, to discuss potential replacements for him when the time arrived. "I might be jumping the gun a bit," he told Sharisse, "because we're not scheduled to leave anytime soon."

"Not at all," she said. "Planning ahead helps smooth the transition when that time comes."

"You won't replace me, will you?" Tyrell asked, somewhat sheepishly.

"Not until you're ready to go," Sharisse said, laughing. "Let's think about who might succeed you and what we need to do to help that person be ready. Any suggestions?"

"Briana's an excellent charge nurse, though she's only been out of school a year or two."

Sharisse jotted down Briana's name. "Anyone else?"

"Olga is good, too. Experienced, but she sometimes rubs people the wrong way."

"Could she be counseled to improve?"

"It hasn't helped so far. But Parker, a part-time nurse, might work out. She's a retired Army nurse. The others go to her with questions when she's on duty."

"So we have two people who could be promoted. Why don't you give each of them some opportunities for leadership, such as serving as charge nurse or committee chair, and evaluate their progress."

"I'm so relieved," Tyrell said. "I like the unit and the work. I wouldn't want to leave you or them without the best help."

"By the time you're ready to leave," Sharisse said, "I'm sure we'll have at least one prepared candidate."

16

Leaving Your Legacy

You only live once—but if you work it right, once is enough.

JOE E. LEWIS

In this chapter, you will learn:

- How you have already created a legacy
- What are ways to leave your legacy
- How to continue to contribute
- How to create a record of your life

LEAVING YOUR LEGACY

Just because you leave your position or retire from paid employment doesn't mean that you can no longer contribute to nursing and health care. You have knowledge and experience to share. You may be financially comfortable and able to contribute some portion of funds to causes you consider deserving. You are entering the next phase of your life.

What Is Your Legacy?

Your legacy is the work you have done, patients you have helped, colleagues you've supported, students you've taught, and everything you have done over the course of your career. You are leaving a legacy every day. Everything you do leaves some result behind. Programs you've presented, committees chaired, people you've educated, community service given, and contributions to your family, spouse, parents, children, and friends: everything you are and have been is a legacy.

Consider Your Past Contributions

You may be surprised at the legacy you are leaving and what you have already contributed. Everything you've done counts. (Go to Learning Activity 1 at the end of this chapter to uncover your legacy.)

For the Novice Nurse

Thinking about preparing your successors is about as relevant to you as planning your retirement. You know it will happen someday, but you can't think about that now. Your career has just begun. You can use this content, however, to guide your future. Here's how to do it: write a letter to your older self. Thank yourself for the work done, the contributions you've made, and the legacy you've left. You may be surprised at all you've accomplished! The next step is to think about how you can make it come true.

Good luck!

PLANNING FOR YOUR FUTURE

Now that you've assessed your legacy at this point in time, consider a plan for your future. Contributing your time, your talents, and your money are ways you can continue to add to your legacy.

Contributing Your Time

You have a wealth of experiences and may have the time to share what you've learned. Today, few people are retiring completely. Phased retirement is becoming the norm rather than the exception. People are continuing to work beyond the typical retirement age in their original field, part-time in another area, or volunteering their services in organizations they value and where their expertise is needed.

For people who have been actively involved in their profession, leaving paid employment may be a considerable loss. Time is no longer structured, and built-in opportunities to interact with colleagues no longer exist. Finding ways to contribute your time to activities you enjoy is a way to share your knowledge and continue to garner satisfaction from the work you do.

Contributing Your Talents

Some nurses find that becoming involved in health policy issues, at either the local or national level, is a way to share their expertise, connect with colleagues, and keep up with the changes in nursing. Redesigning health care, as recommended by the Institute of Medicine (2010) and radically changing nursing education, as the Carnegie Foundation (Benner et al., 2009) advises is challenging nursing practice and education. Serving on a local nursing school's advisory board, for example, is be one way to contribute.

You have learned much over the course of a career, and you could share your knowledge with the general public as well. As you know, the public is mostly uninformed about the work nurses do and the vital role nurses play in health care. You can change that lack of knowledge in formal and informal ways. Remember that you learned how we represent nursing in everything we do. As a respected member of the nursing profession, you have an unparalleled opportunity to affect the public's perception of nursing.

Here are just a few examples of ways you might contribute now:

- Write an op-ed piece for your local newspaper.
- Volunteer at a hospital or food kitchen.
- Review a book about health care for your local paper or professional organization.
- Serve on committees or boards of nursing or community groups.

Even if you think you've done all you care to do, you may be drawn into such activities as writing a letter to the editor of your local paper after you read an article that stimulates you to respond. You may be active in your church, synagogue, mosque, or community organization and find that your talents are called upon in their activities. Your family and friends may ask your advice from time to time. Accept your role as a senior advisor. You have much to offer.

CONTRIBUTING YOUR MONEY In addition to sharing your time and talents, consider contributing another resource: your money. Interestingly, nurses seem reluctant to give money even to causes they support (see link to "Giving" in the end-of-chapter Web Resources section). Why do you think that is? Granted, we have less to give than others, but we can give some. Still, nurses seem reluctant.

It may be that our heritage as nurses and (predominantly) women has prepared us to give our talents and time but seldom our money. Women today have experienced professional success and have control of their own money. Nurses, too, can decide how and where to give their money.

Giving money is another way to leave a legacy for the future. Donating to an endowment that will live on in perpetuity gives us the satisfaction of knowing that our contribution will make a difference long after we are no longer living. Sometimes, though, we give because we feel pressured to do so. A friend asks for a donation for a just cause or our employer wants 100 percent participation in the local United Way campaign, and we acquiesce. There is a better way to target our giving and know that our money is going to the places we consider the most worthy.

Here are some suggestions for planning your giving:

- Consider your giving as falling into two categories: periodic giving during your lifetime and your final gift.
- Designate a portion of your annual income for charitable giving.
- Divide your annual gift among a few organizations based on your commitment to their mission and their need.
- Review your plan yearly and adjust it as your circumstances and their needs change.
- Arrange for your assets to be distributed upon your death (yes, it is inevitable) and explore the many options for planned giving.
- Encourage your children or other relatives to give by designating a portion of your estate to charitable and other organizations.
- Tell your family about your decisions so that there are no surprises later.

There are several benefits to this planning. First, you know how much you are prepared to give each year and can budget accordingly. Second, you are better prepared to decline other unplanned giving requests. Finally, you are teaching your family that they are not entitled to all your assets (actually, they aren't "entitled" to any of it). They can learn from your example, and their potential future gifts would be another legacy from you.

Recording Your Life

Many people choose to create a history of their family, their life, or their work to share with others now or in the future. Creating a life history can benefit you as well. Taking time to recall events, people, and circumstances helps us to accept our past and to face our future with satisfaction. Providing a record of our life and experiences is another way we can leave our legacy.

You can write your history or record it in video or audio. Put it in a safe place (don't rely on just a file on your computer) and let someone know where it is.

What You Know Now

You have learned that your legacy is everything you have done over the course of your professional and personal life. You know, too, that you have many opportunities to continue to contribute to your legacy with your time, your talents, and your money. You have learned that you can organize your charitable giving to benefit organizations now and in the future and that you can teach your family the value of giving. You know how to create a record of your life for yourself as well as for others.

Your legacy lives on in the work you have done and the person you are. Be proud of it.

Tools for Leaving Your Legacy

1. Consider all the ways in which you are leaving a legacy.
2. Recognize your unique talents and consider ways in which you might continue to contribute.
3. Think about how and where you want your money to go now and in the future.
4. Arrange for your financial goals to be met.

Learning Activities

1. Evaluate your past contributions. Make a list of each job you have had, including volunteer positions in nursing, health care, or community organizations. Under each position, list how you contributed or what was accomplished during your involvement. You won't have done it all, but you will have contributed to the collective effort. Count everything.

   Take some time to ponder the many contributions you've made. Celebrate your accomplishments with something special for yourself.
2. Consider writing a history of your life. Start by jotting down events, dates, and people as you recall them without trying to put anything in order yet. Later, you can sort these by date or year. Occasionally, get out your list and add anything that comes to mind. You might try adding to it at the end of the year, but don't make this an onerous task. Just do as much as you want to at a time.

   Put your list somewhere you can find it easily. See what you think of the next time you get it out.
3. Think about what you'd like to contribute in the future. Jot down everything that comes to mind without thinking about how it could happen. Don't edit it now. Put your list aside for now.

   Come back to your list sometime later. Decide what you would like to do most. Build a plan for accomplishing your first priority and one or two more if you want. Think about the value of what you are planning. When you've accomplished your goal, what might be the result?

   Start on your plan!

References

Institute of Medicine (2010). *The future of nursing: Leading change, advancing health.* Retrieved October 15, 2010, from http://www.thefutureofnursing.org/IOM-Report

Benner, P., Sutphen, M., Leonard, V., & Day, L. (2009). *Educating nurses: A call for radical transformation.* San Francisco: Jossey-Bass.

Web Resource

Sullivan, E. J. Giving. *Journal of Professional Nursing, 16*(6). Retrieved April 15, 2011, from http://www.eleanorsullivan.com/pdf/giving.pdf

CASE STUDY

A Nurse Leaves Her Legacy

Before she retired, Clarissa worked in numerous positions at a major teaching hospital. She'd started on the medical floor, moved to the ICU, worked for a time in the ER, and finished her career as a case manager. Clarissa knew she'd made a difference in many patients' lives. She often saw former patients or their family members when they visited at the hospital, and many remembered her help.

Clarissa looked into retirement. Financially, she could maintain her lifestyle and enjoy additional benefits. She wanted to travel, to spend time with her family, and to volunteer at a halfway house for abused women. Working in the emergency room, she'd seen how their lives were devastated by abuse, and she wanted to help. Also, she wanted to contribute her expertise to a local nonprofit organization.

Knowing she would miss her job and her colleagues, Clarissa made a plan before finalizing her retirement. She found several resources that reflected her interests. She joined a travel group, signed up with local genealogy organization, and set up an appointment with the nursing director at a homeless shelter. Before her retirement date, she'd already met with several people who shared similar interests and scheduled more in the future. Clarissa said goodbye to friends and colleagues and embarked on the next phase of her life.

After enjoying her new life for a while, Clarissa reflected on how to allocate her financial resources. For final distribution of her assets, she saw an attorney, established a revocable trust, assigned a nephew to serve as her executor and hold power of attorney for health care decisions, and drew up a will. Although it was not easy to think about, she knew that taking care of her final arrangements was a way to relieve her family of that burden.

For giving on an annual basis, she thought about the charities that interested her. She wanted to help future nurses, so she set aside a specific amount to donate to her alma mater for nursing scholarships. She'd been volunteering at the homeless shelter, so she allocated an amount to be donated to it. A nurse friend worked at an organization that served people with disabilities, and she allotted a portion each year for them. Finally, she set aside some discretionary money to give away as she saw needs occur during the year.

Clarissa had successfully transitioned from a working nurse to a life as satisfying and fulfilling as her career had been.

Plus, she had a great deal of fun!

APPENDIX

Ten Little-Known Secrets for Success

1. Do each job the best you can.
2. Make others look good.
3. Take chances.
4. You are what you say you are.
5. Say what you mean; mean what you say.
6. Watch others.
7. Learn the rules.
8. Know what fits for you.
9. Find a cause greater than yourself.
10. Keep your eye on the future.

INDEX

P

Q

R